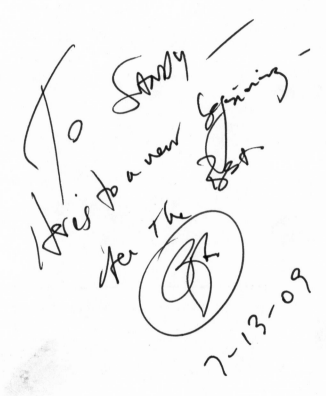

To Sandy —

Here's to a new Beginning —

for The

7-13-09

Health For The Whole Family – For Life!

The Great Health Heist

Recapture Your Family's Health

Safely, Naturally and Effectively

Using Nutrition Response Testing[SM]

Paul J. Rosen, J.D., L.Ac.

Warren Publishing, Inc.

Cornelius, NC

The Great Health Heist

Published by Warren Publishing, Inc.

ISBN 1-886057-18-4

Library of Congress Control Number: 2007933960

Printed in the United States of America

They Stole Your Health –

Now Take It Back!

"POWERFUL INFORMATION......... A MUST READ FOR ANYONE CONCERNED WITH THEIR HEALTH AND THAT OF FUTURE GENERATIONS!"

"THE GREAT HEALTH HEIST GOES RIGHT TO THE HEART OF WHAT'S CAUSING OUR CURRENT HEALTH CARE CRISIS!"

~ Joseph J. Teff D.C.

* * * * *

"Quite simply Paul Rosen's book is compelling. It exposes the myths within and about the current health care system and explains why we are really sick. The time has come for people to know the truth. No longer do you have to accept the "non-answer" responses from established medicine, which often leave you scratching your head, or feeling somehow the failure to address your condition is your fault. Paul Rosen proves there is hope. This book will allow you to once and for all take charge of your health."

~ Lori Puskar, D.C.

* * * * *

"If you are one of the millions of people who knows that their health is not what it could be then you won't be able to put Paul Rosen's book down. Nutrition Response Testing, as explained in the book, is a tool for health analysis that has been as much a boon to health care professionals as to those seeking better health. Doctors were as lost as their patients in trying to find the root causes of disease, but now there is a specialized system that quickly and easily lays out the path to wellness."

~ *Jeannette Birnbach, D.C., M.S., C.C.N*

What Enthusiastic Patients Are Saying:

"My daughter, Sara, age 11, had stomach pain for over a year to the point of vomiting and uncontrollable shaking. The doctors diagnosed her with Functional Abdominal Pain [but had no answers]. After approximately 1½ months on the program, my daughter has had an incredible turn around in her health, which is reflected in every part of her life. Her little vivacious attitude is back. She is able to sleep at night with no vomiting or shaking, and no pain in her stomach...."

~ *L.S.*

* * * * *

"I had a dry cough that was embarrassing. I craved sweets and wanted to lose weight. I squeezed in Curves once a day for one month and managed to lose [only] 5 pounds. [But my symptoms remained]. [After being evaluated using Nutrition Response Testing and being on the program], my cough disappeared unless I ate foods I wasn't supposed to. What's more, I've lost 10 [more] pounds, my sugar cravings AND I've had compliments about my [new] appearance."

~ *V.S.*

* * * * *

"I was always tired [diagnosed with chronic fatigue], caught many colds that would last for weeks, had knee pain, low energy, and felt run down. Now my energy is solid. I am able to hike for six to eight miles without the use of hiking poles. I haven't had any more colds or knee pain, and am sleeping well. I am feeling very healthy and strong."

~ L.H.

* * * * *

"I was not able to quit smoking. I have tried for many years. Now, I'm very happy to say that I've gone a whole week without a cigarette and plan on not having one again."

~ D.C.

* * * * *

"I used to have a headache almost every day or every other day. During the last five years or so I started experiencing migraines also. I had no idea what was causing them and was starting to get concerned that something serious might be wrong with me. I started on the [Nutrition Response Testing] program and within a week the headaches were gone."

~ R.S.

This book is dedicated to all of us, men, women and children alike, who are trying to handle our most pressing health concerns by sticking to our guns in the knowledge that drugs and surgery are not the holy grail of healthcare. We have taken control of our own health by opening our minds to new approaches and being willing to make the necessary changes in our lives to achieve positive results using safe, natural and effective treatment.

An excerpt from

The Great Health Heist

*In his book **Death By Prescription**, Raymond Strand, M.D. is emphatic that drugs are a "clear and present danger" to our health. He further states that each individual is ultimately responsible for making an informed decision regarding his or her own health.*

Reliance on medical doctors and the healthcare system is simply not good enough anymore. Drugs, even when properly prescribed, are the fourth-rated cause of death in the United States. Then there is the role our government plays in the form of the FDA.

The first effort to protect the public's food supply – our food supply – from additives, colors and potential poisons came in the form of the Food and Drug Act on June 30, 1906. The FDA's predecessor, the Bureau of Chemistry, was charged with oversight and enforcement.

To the chagrin of the Bureau's father, Dr. Harvey Wiley, his efforts to enforce the law not only met with resistance but also resulted in his dismissal and replacement by a food industry "mouthpiece."

Worse yet, despite a Supreme Court ruling for consumers, those in charge of enforcement sidestepped the law via nuance and slight of hand, exposing millions to health risks and leaving the Food and Drug Act toothless. Fast-forward to today when adulterated foods, including exposure to thousands of potentially dangerous chemicals, are the norm.

*Although locating a copy of Dr. Wiley's book, **History of a Crime**, requires a countrywide search (and a bit of luck), I would be happy to supply anyone with its conclusion. With the food supply in jeopardy and personal health at risk, drugs would surely come to the rescue.*

Could we rely on the FDA for protection?

As of 2003, according to Dr. Strand, the FDA, in charge of oversight of the safety and effectiveness of drugs, had only 65 trained professionals with advanced degrees to monitor thousands of drugs and hundreds of drug companies. Moreover, he wrote, "more than 50% of the money to fund the FDA is provided by the pharmaceutical industry in the form of 'user fees'." 50%! As you can see, the fox is guarding the hen house! Can you say conflict of interest?!?

Worse yet, within the last decade legislation has relaxed the rules for companies bringing drugs to market. "Fast Tracking," as it is referred to, has unleashed a slew of drugs on the market whose safety and effectiveness have been compromised. Dr. Strand's book is a must-read before deciding to take another prescription medication.

In the face of all this bad news, what can you do? Simply, WAKE UP, look in the mirror and take control of your own health.

Fortunately for you and me there is technology available to handle most health problems safely, naturally and effectively without the onerous risks of drugs.

It is called Nutrition Response Testing.

Nutrition Response Testing can solve the riddle of many chronic functional illnesses. These illnesses include chronic fatigue, fibromyalgia, migraines, allergies, chronic pain, PMS, hot flashes, night sweats, constipation, IBS, high blood pressure and many others.

This near-miraculous method of evaluation unlocks the innate power of the perpetual healing machine called the human body, the most powerful healing tool on the planet.

Table of Contents

Foreword

I have been helping people improve their health for more than four decades using safe, natural and effective alternatives to drugs and surgery. But along the way, conditions that once responded successfully seemed resistant to the tools I had relied on for so long. I wanted to know why.

Suddenly, during one of the most productive periods in my life, I began to experience life-threatening health problems of my own. I reached out to my old colleague and mentor, Dr. Lester Bryman, D.C., C.D.N. This wonderful man not only helped me restore my health but he introduced me to a breakthrough technology in healing using a highly effective nutritional program.

With my health on the rebound and with a fervent desire to share my positive health experiences, Dr. Bryman and I took this technology that was based on earlier developments, and raised it to a new high. We now call it "Nutrition Response Testing℠."

Still we had a much larger vision. We realized that in order to reach as many people as possible, we needed (1) to train other practitioners in the technical aspects of Nutrition Response Testing and (2) to show them how to grow and administer their own successful nutrition practices. To that end, we developed a powerful training program that would inspire and enable other like-minded practitioners to attain the same exciting results we achieved for our patients. We are dedicated to helping all willing practitioners build truly effective nutritional practices that answer the needs of the growing number of people seeking safe, natural and effective solutions to their health problems. I am proud to say that today we are achieving just that.

Dedicated health-care providers who have taken the knowledge Dr. Bryman and I have accumulated over decades of clinical experience are now helping countless thousands of people throughout the United States. This has expanded into a much needed and very much appreciated "win, win, win" situation for all concerned: the patient, the practitioner and the community. The future of healthy living looks brighter and brighter for our children, our grandchildren and for generations to come.

Paul Rosen's book, *The Great Health Heist*, captures the essence of this 'triple win' scenario. He reveals the unethical behaviors of those "authorities" upon whom we have previously relied, but who have repeatedly let us down. These people have deceived us using both misinformation and misdeeds with, too often, harmful results. He calls upon everyone, whether patient or health-care provider, to take back a higher level of responsibility for their own health as well as that of their family, friends and communities.

If you're concerned about your health or simply want to get healthier and maintain your health at the highest possible level, come aboard and join the thousands of others who know the future today with Nutrition Response Testing. It is my sincerest hope that you will breathe new vitality into your life in the same manner in which it was breathed into mine, and that you gain the knowledge needed to maintain it for a healthy and vital future.

Freddie Ulan, D.C., C.C.N.
Clearwater, Florida

Preface

"Physician, Heal Thyself"

Although I am a licensed acupuncturist and not a medical doctor, I believe the phrase "physician, heal thyself" clearly applies to all practitioners of the healing arts. I, like you, desire to stay healthy, active and able to take care of loved ones. Before 1996, I ate well (or so I thought), took vitamins, had regular checkups, exercised regularly and believed I knew what I was doing. I was introduced to whole-food nutrition as a teenager and later in my life studied oriental medicine and became a practitioner. But in 1996 everything went terribly wrong.

While waiting for a plane home after a fishing trip in Idaho, my heartbeat became irregular. I found myself in the emergency room of the local hospital. After being examined, I was told I was dehydrated and was released. Upon returning home, I experienced deep fatigue, I couldn't get from the bed to a chair without assistance, had continuing heart irregularities, panic attacks and feelings of suffocation.

The list went on and on. I reduced my hours at work and saw every kind of health practitioner: homeopath, osteopath, acupuncturist/herbalist, chiropractor, etc. Each discipline helped a little. But years passed – I had reached a plateau. I was stuck!

Then, in 2003, a friend introduced me to Dr. Freddie Ulan and the work he called Nutrition Response Testing℠. Dr. Ulan evaluated me and found I had thyroid exhaustion, digestive enzyme deficiencies and an immune challenge. He put me on a health improvement program of whole-food supplements and dietary changes.

Within weeks, I began to feel better. I hadn't felt that good in years! Amazed, I began to increase my professional studies, took courses, did research, and read extensively about nutrition and Nutrition Response Testing.

I applied what I learned to my acupuncture patients who were not progressing and the results were undeniable. I was able to crack the toughest cases. I emailed Dr. Ulan and asked him to teach me everything he knew. Fortunately for me, he did just that.

So, for all of you who have suffered more than your share with chronic health conditions such as weight problems, allergies, fatigue, chronic pain, chronic infections, repeated colds or flu, migraines, headaches, insomnia, PMS, menopause or the endless list of other conditions, do what I did – find the missing piece that solves your health concern.

For those of you who have no symptoms but know the value of preventative health, stop guessing. With Nutrition Response Testing, your precise nutritional needs will be revealed. And don't confuse lack of symptoms with good health, as many people do. Every human body has special requirements and this technology allows us to listen to its requests. Nutrition Response Testing is painless, powerful and personalized. Only safe, natural and effective tools are used for treatment.

Thousands of people are feeling better today.

Isn't it your turn?

I invite you to join me on this incredible journey.

Isn't it time you took more control over your health?

Aren't you ready to make a change?

Health Heist Handbook:

Each discipline helped a little. But years passed –
I had reached a plateau. I was stuck!

PAUL J. ROSEN, J.D., L.AC.

Acknowledgments

I am grateful to the following people who gave me life, saved my life, continue to sustain my life and make it possible for me to serve others in a way I could only have dreamed of. Gratitude is the reason to serve, and service is the means by which we are fulfilled and help others to fulfill themselves.

I want to thank my parents, Madalyn and Stanley Q; my teachers Swami Chetanananda, Rudi and Bhagawan Nityananda; Drs. Freddie Ulan, Lester Bryman, Bong Dal Kim and Richard Tan. There have been many others, too, who have been willing to share what they know in furtherance of my growth; you know who you are and I thank you.

Of course, if it weren't for the efforts of Rusty Fisher, my editor, with his experience, encouragement and guidance, the book would not have been completed. Thank you. Regarding copyediting, thank you Beth, Jeannette and my wife.

9

Finally, to my wife Cheryl, whose love and companionship have made and continue to make it possible for me to do whatever I'm doing on our journey together. Thank you, my dearest darling!

Part 1

Is Your Health in Crisis?

Chapter 1

Do You Feel Like Your Health's Been Stolen?
TAKE IT BACK!

Heist *(n)* 1.) to commit robbery on 2.) TO STEAL

How did you feel when you woke up this morning?

It's a simple question, but I'll ask it again: How did you feel when you woke up this morning? Often when I ask this question, my new patients immediately start in with the excuses:

- "Well, not so good, but it's my own fault. I didn't sleep well because I missed that deadline at work and tossed and turned thinking about it…"

- "Well, I had a headache, but I always get one when I use the wrong pillow so really it's my own fault..."
- "Not great, but better than when I'm hungover..."
- "Okay, I mean, for the most part. I shouldn't have had that bowl of ice cream at midnight. I guess I should know better by now..."
- "Great! Super! I mean, except for my back. And my neck. And my feet..."

Sound familiar? Well, forget the fact that all of these answers, and the hundreds of other excuses I hear every day, point to less than optimum health. There is another, just as important issue at hand: Why do we feel the need to make excuses for how we feel in the morning?

Would it be so wrong to admit we feel lousy? Un-rested? Un-healthy? Un-satisfied? Why must we constantly deny our true feelings and cover up for our own poor health? Is it because we know, deep down, that we should feel better? Is it because it's been so long since we've felt good?

Think back to your childhood and how you greeted each day. Okay, rewind, do over: Think back to your childhood and how you greeted each **non-school** day. My friends and I would literally bound out of bed and onto the street each morning, bright and eager for a game of catch or street hockey, or a treasure hunt or marathon bike trip through town.

Our parents would literally have to shove food down our throats on the way out the door. There was no such thing as a snooze button, over-the-counter stimulant or steaming cup of coffee; all we needed were sneakers, skivvies and sunshine to start the day – and even those were optional!

It didn't matter if we had pneumonia or a broken arm, our thoughts were on getting out of bed and out into the world, eager for that next adventure that lay just over the distant horizon.

What happened along the way? How did we get to the point where it takes six stabs at the snooze button, a few pills, several cups of coffee, a scalding shower and several more cups of coffee just to greet the day?

And you haven't even reached the breakfast table yet!

What if I told you that you could retrieve that childhood feeling of innocence, energy, fun and purity again? What if I told you there is a better way to give your body what it needs – when it needs it – that doesn't come out of a prescription bottle, over the counter box, forty-dollar tube or drive-thru window?

The energy is right there at your fingertips; you just need to reach for it.

The truth is out there; you just need to uncover it.

The knowledge is inside you; you just need to rediscover it.

The best part is you don't need to learn anything new, but only UN-learn what teachers, scientists, researchers, faddists, the media and other so-called experts have "taught" you over the years. So think of this not as a how-to book, but more as a how-**not**-to book!

The fact of the matter is that your health didn't dissipate, fracture, dissolve or dry up. You didn't misplace your health, forget about it, neglect it (well maybe you did) or even ignore it. Your health wasn't lost – it was **STOLEN**!

That's right. Additive-inventors, pseudo-scientists, "health" reporters, diet books, fitness magazines, even vitamin supplement advertisers and corporate conglomerates – and let's not forget the prescription drug folks – stole your health right out from under you.

They didn't wear masks, but they certainly crept into your life just the same. They didn't use guns, but instead chose words, statistics, slim models, appealing photography and packaging to rob you of your common sense. They didn't drive a getaway car, but they're sure enough laughing – all the way to the bank!

Bottom line: they stole your health – now take it back!

The Great Health Heist is no exaggeration; it's the truth. And the truth really will set you free; free from the laundry list of afflictions that stress you out, weigh you down, bind you up and make you feel less than whole.

In this book I will explain not only what I mean by *The Great Health Heist*, but also how to **take your health back** using a very simple tool that can literally make you feel like a kid again.

I started this section with a question, so it's only fitting I end it the same way. Actually, I have a few questions for you. Here goes:

- Are you tired of making excuses for how you feel in the morning?
- Are you ready to stop making excuses – and start living?
- Are you ready to feel like a kid again?
- Are you tired of having your health stolen by drugs, additives, fast food, junk food and just plain *bad* food?
- Are you ready to take your health back?

If the answer to all of the above is "yes," then let me introduce you to the people, pharmaceuticals, organizations, additives, myths and outright lies that stole your health.

Welcome, friends, to *The Great Health Heist*!

Health Heist Handbook:

You didn't misplace your health, forget about it, neglect it or even ignore it. On second thought, maybe you were an accomplice BUT your health wasn't lost – it was STOLEN!

Chapter 2

How We Got Into This Fix

Our current health crisis didn't happen overnight, nor are we entirely innocent when it comes to committing often negligent, and occasionally purposeful, criminal acts against our own bodies.

In fact, you might even say we are accomplices in our own health crisis.

They say we do better when we know better, but for some reason this and every other well-meaning truism just seems to fly out the window when it comes to eating. Don't believe me? How often have you nodded your head over some great wisdom in the latest health journal or written yourself a note about avoiding trans fats or fried foods, all while waiting in the jammed drive-thru lane at your favorite fast-food joint?

The bad news is your health is still in crisis – or soon will be.

The good news is you're far from alone. Despite record sales of vitamin supplements, the overall health of people today continues to decline. No matter how many warnings regarding the plague of processed foods, people keep eating glazed doughnuts and washing them down with triple lattes.

Is there any wonder why chronic diseases including obesity, diabetes and heart disease continue to climb? Even real-life demonstrations of rapid health decline, such as those reported in the 2003 documentary *"Super Size Me,"* don't seem to slow people down!

Part of the problem is our love-hate relationship with the popular media, and how we trust some blindly even as we don't trust others at all. Our main issue, then, becomes one of trust.

Who to trust?

What to trust?

When to trust?

Case in point: I was reading the paper the other day and, lo and behold, I discovered a group financed by the processed food industry called The Center for Consumer Freedom. Billing themselves as a "nonprofit coalition of restaurants, food companies, and consumers working together to promote personal responsibility and protect consumer choices," this organization was formed in 1995 with money from Philip Morris, now known as Altria, to fight bans on smoking in restaurants and bars.

They argue that obesity isn't as bad as everyone says it is because the stats are overblown, advocating that there are only 112,000 deaths attributed to obesity each year instead of the 400,000 reported by the Centers for Disease Control. This group goes on to conclude that there is no epidemic and therefore "the obesity thing" is blown "way out of proportion!" What else would you expect from a proponent of the $500 billion a year counterfeit food industry?

Regardless of whether obesity is directly linked to the premature deaths of 400,000 people each year or 112,000 – or even 112 people for that matter, there is no argument that health-related problems from obesity cost states and their taxpayers $60-75 billion; money that could be spent on things like improving education for students and displaced workers or finding alternative sources of energy.

But as one who insists on looking for points of agreement, I find both this group and myself urging the following philosophy: Don't blame the cow for soggy cornflakes. (My words, not theirs.) In other words, just because processed food is available doesn't mean you have to eat it. I know, I know, it sort of sounds like the "guns don't kill people, people kill people" argument made by the National Rifle Association. But if the shoe fits...

It all boils down to personal accountability. In other words, it's *your* responsibility to know what's best for you, to the best of your ability. This does not mean taking a crash course in nutrition or physiology and it doesn't mean you should do it on your own. But by now even the most casual observer of current events knows the bare bones arguments against obesity, high cholesterol, elevated blood pressure, hydrogenated fat and processed foods.

I asked earlier who you could trust. The answer: trust begins with someone who will tell you the truth. And in this case, truth refers to an approach that works.

If you're the type of person who knows that what you eat has a good chance of resulting in poor health sooner rather than later and you continue to eat it anyway, then I guess you get what you deserve. But if you're sick and tired of being sick and tired and are ready to find the "missing piece" that will resolve your health concerns, then get ready for some eye-opening discoveries.

Health Heist Handbook:

Is there any wonder why chronic diseases, including obesity, diabetes and heart disease, continue to climb?

Chapter 3

Name That Disease

Currently, reality shows are very popular. Well, here's one for you: Let's call it "Name That Disease." If Americans continue to eat processed foods at the current rate, our immune systems will become so compromised that eventually we will barely be able to withstand the common cold. Oh, wait a minute. This is already true for many of you, isn't it?

In the 1940s, Dr. Francis M. Pottenger, Jr., a doctor who researched cures for tuberculosis, pioneered the use of adrenal extracts and nutrition in the treatment of fatigue. His research made an additional startling discovery; while feeding his experimental subjects – cats – processed (or cooked) food, serious health conditions manifested, including deformities, lack of physical coordination and infertility. Moreover, within three generations the cats were so arthritic, they were unable to walk to the front of their cages to feed themselves.

Today the leading cause of disability in our country is arthritis. Coincidence or certainty? We all eat processed or cooked foods. Whether it's zapped under a heat lamp at some fast-food joint or flash frozen in some factory, processed food is an integral part of our daily diet.

The scary part is that Dr. Pottenger's findings support the proposition that eating nutritionally bankrupt food can alter genetic attributes. Moreover, these altered traits can be passed on to future generations. Did you hear that correctly? Eating a daily diet heavy in processed food not only puts your own health at risk, but the health of your children and *their* children too! This is headline news, but I'm certain you've never heard of Dr. Pottenger or his findings.

Another groundbreaking physician you've probably never heard of is Dr. Weston Price. Dr. Price, in his treatise ***Nutrition and Physical Degeneration***, demonstrated without a doubt that nutritional deficiencies caused disease. In fact, there were many great men between 1900 and 1950 who contributed to understanding the connection between processed, or nutritionally bankrupt foods and poor health.

None were more important than Dr. Royal Lee, the founder of both the Lee Foundation for Nutritional Research in 1941 and the Vitamin Products Company, now known as Standard Process. Standard Process's whole raw food concentrates remain the mainstay in the tool chests of the most effective practitioners of nutrition today.

Despite the work of dedicated, passionate physicians like Pottenger, Price and Lee, the national health crisis continued to churn on with all the momentum of a tidal wave of grease and fat. Never letting science and facts stand in the way of progress, the food, pharmaceutical and tobacco industries have for decades co-opted the healthcare agenda by misdirecting and feeding the public half-truths or outright falsehoods to entice them to create and then satisfy their cravings.

In his book **Empty Harvest**, Dr. Bernard Jensen displayed advertisements for cigarettes from 1937 that touted their benefits for – get this – "digestive function." Moreover, sugar was trumpeted as "healthy calories" and "an effective way to lose weight" (1955). Pharmaceutical companies simply promoted the use of poisons (drugs) for the treatment of conditions that are, in fact, symptoms of malnutrition; for example, arthritis and diabetes.

Today, the tobacco example seems ludicrous in the face of what we now know or, perhaps I should say, what we have finally accepted. And yet how will future generations react when they see 500-calorie shakes billed as "nutritional supplements" and flash-frozen, pre-packaged, preservative-injected, processed meat, vegetables and desserts billed as "healthy choices?" No doubt they will snicker just as we snicker over tobacco ads from the 1930s.

So what does that say about us?

Want to know why your health continues to slip away? The following description of events should give you a clue: Based on their unethical conduct, cigarette companies have been successfully sued for fraudulently misrepresenting their products by states clearly benefiting from their sale by collecting billions of dollars in taxes. But in order to collect the judgment against the companies, the states allow them to stay in business and supply a willing public (who continues to risk serious health problems), which in turn drives up healthcare costs for all of us. This same public then sues the cigarette companies, hoping to collect millions for failing to warn of health hazards despite being warned as early as the 1960s.

Oh, what a tangled web we weave!

And then there is sugar. Studies show that refined cane sugar saps the body of precious minerals. Dextrose, a sugar derived from corn (or, in some instances, wood chips) and one of the most widely used sweeteners in the food industry as far back as the early to mid-1900s, is shown to produce diabetes in laboratory animal studies. In fact, research shows not only that cancer cells cannot survive without a good supply of sugar, but that technologies like PET scanners require sugar (in the form of glucose solutions) to detect cancerous tumors.

Another highly refined sweetener, high fructose corn syrup, or HFCS, has become the sweetener of choice for the food industry since the mid-1970s. Coincidently, incidents of obesity have skyrocketed. Despite hundreds of billions of dollars spent and the creation of a countrywide network of research, cancer continues to challenge heart disease as the number one killer. New cases of diabetes have increased over 50% between 1997 and 2004.

Despite the clear connection between refined sweeteners and disease, including the known addictive quality of sugar, the food industry continues to saturate their products with these ingredients. Do you still believe that they desire to nourish and support your health?

Unfortunately, the pharmaceutical industry is equally disappointing, using the media to hype a so-called "caring" advertising theme while undermining your health and looting your pocketbook. In her book **The Truth about the Drug Companies**: *How They Deceive Us and What to Do about It,* Marcia Angell, M.D., reveals that "Big Pharma" has become an out-of-control bull (my words, not hers) masquerading as educators and researchers, using their power, influence and money to stretch out their monopolies and deceive the public into believing that their "me, too" drugs are the next miracle.

Dr. Angell's suggestions are three-fold:

1) Ask your prescribing doctor what evidence there is that a drug is better than some other approach to treatment. Are the benefits of this drug worth the side effects, expense and risk of interactions with other drugs?

2) Ask your senators and representatives in Congress if they receive campaign contributions from the pharmaceutical industry and, if so, how much.

3) Pay no attention to direct-to-consumer ads for prescription drugs. In other words, WAKE UP, look in the mirror and take control of your health.

So, are drugs really the answer? The more symptomatic conditions we experience, the more the drug companies find ways to suppress them.

Got allergies? Take Allerest.

Got acid reflux? Take Prilosec.

Got a headache or arthritis? Take Vioxx.

Should the symptom disappear, hooray! You're happy (for now), but are you any healthier? Of course not! All these drugs do for a person is turn off the "check engine lights," leaving the cause unidentified, and you more vulnerable to future disease. This ultimately foolish strategy costs every man, woman and child in the country more than $6,711 per year in medical costs, and the figure is rising.

Despite the fact that we spend more money on healthcare every year, the overall health of Americans continues to slide. The World Health Organization (WHO) ranks United States 37th among current industrialized nations in providing healthcare for its citizens.

It's become very clear that many drugs disguise the slippery slope toward degenerative disease!

Health Heist Handbook:

Dr. Pottenger's findings support the proposition that genetic attributes can be altered by eating nutritionally bankrupt food – and those inferior alterations can be passed on to your children!

Chapter 4

A Clear and Present Danger

In his book **Death by Prescription**, Raymond Strand, M.D. is emphatic that drugs are a "clear and present danger" to our health. He further states (in so many words) that we, as individuals, are ultimately responsible for making informed decisions regarding our own health.

Reliance on medical doctors and the healthcare system is simply not good enough anymore. Drugs, even when properly prescribed, are the fourth-rated cause of death in the United States. And then there is the role our government plays in the form of the FDA.

The FDA, in charge of overseeing the safety and effectiveness of drugs, has only 65 trained professionals with advanced degrees to monitor thousands of drugs and hundreds of drug companies. In addition, more than 50% of the money funding the FDA comes from the pharmaceutical industry – 50%. That's right! The fox is guarding the hen house! Can you say conflict of interest?!?

Worse yet, legislation within the last decade has relaxed the rules for companies bringing drugs to market. "Fast Tracking," as it is referred to, has unleashed a slew of drugs on the market whose safety and effectiveness have been compromised. Dr. Strand's book should definitely be a must-read before you decide to take another prescription medication.

In the face of all this bad news, what can you do? Simple: WAKE UP, look in the mirror and take control of your own health. Fortunately there is technology available to handle most health problems safely, naturally and effectively without the onerous risks of drugs.

It is called Nutrition Response Testing.

Nutrition Response Testing can solve the riddle of so many chronic functional illnesses. These illnesses include chronic fatigue, fibromyalgia, migraines, allergies, chronic pain, PMS, hot flashes, night sweats, constipation, IBS, high blood pressure and many others.

This near-miraculous method of evaluation unlocks the innate power of the perpetual healing machine called the human body, the most powerful healing tool on the planet.

Nutrition Response Testing combines knowledge of the autonomic nervous system, which is the body's system that controls all of your vital functions (like heart rate, breathing rate or digestive operations), with the breakthroughs in applied and clinical kinesiology that occurred in the early 1960s. Applied kinesiology has been recognized in this country since at least the early 20th century and is commonly known as muscle testing.

In order to test the autonomic functions of the body, muscles or muscle groups are used in conjunction with known body reflexes. A reflex is an area or point on the body that corresponds to or stimulates another area of the body (like an organ or a gland such as the liver or thyroid). This is the basis upon which reflexology and acupuncture work. In fact, these reflexes often coincide with acupuncture points. They also coincide with dermatomes, or areas of the skin supplied by nerves from the spine. Various means of stimulating these reflexes, including tapping or placing a hand on them, reveal the state of "stress" on the organs and glands, thus giving the practitioner a read on their condition.

The information gathered in this manner is referred to as the innate intelligence of the body; innate as opposed to educated intelligence. What's the difference? Plenty. Innate intelligence refers to that which is inborn and unencumbered. Educated intelligence refers to knowledge that feeds our minds through books and clinical experience.

Muscle testing may be controversial since it flies in the face of Western medicine's reliance on chemistry from blood, urine and stool tests to gather information about the body's condition. But if these tests revealed all there is to know about your condition, and you've probably undergone plenty of them, why are you still suffering? Please don't misread my intentions here. I'm not advocating skipping these tests, but I ask again: What if they don't reveal all there is to know about your condition?

Could it be that something is being missed?

The answer is a resounding **YES**; your "hidden health problem" remains hidden. But there is a technology that can reveal this "missing piece," and muscle testing will open the door to the treasure. Arthur C. Clarke, the renowned science fiction writer, scientist (father of the synchronous earth orbiting of satellites) and Academy Award nominee for *2001: A Space Odyssey*, wrote in his 1962 book *Profiles of the Future* that, "any sufficiently advanced technology is indistinguishable from magic."

As a phenomenon, muscle testing is like gravity, in that gravity operates **whether we believe in it or not**. Therefore, while it is okay to be skeptical, keep an open mind as you read the stories of people just like you who have seen near-miraculous health improvement through Nutrition Response Testing. Just remember that not too long ago in the history of humankind the powers-that-be tried to squash anyone who dared to defy the commonly held belief that the world was flat, not round.

Scientific validation of any theory or test is measured by obtaining duplicatable results, and results are what you deserve. As performed within the context of Nutrition Response Testing, muscle testing has demonstrated its effectiveness and now you can avail yourself of its simplicity. Come and, once and for all, get healthy and stay healthy safely, naturally and effectively with Nutrition Response Testing.

Health Heist Handbook:

In the face of all this bad news, what can you do?
Simple: WAKE UP, look in the mirror and take
control of your own health.

Chapter 5

The Usual Suspects

The promise of good adult health is dependent upon at least two key factors: **good genes** and **good nutrition**. Unfortunately, these factors are no longer equal; nutrition can sway your health in one direction or the other, and not always with an inclination for the better.

Proper nutrition can compensate for negative genetic factors while poor nutrition can overshadow even the most positive genetic traits. Science has already proven that genetic attributes can be affected by nutritional deficiencies. No matter how you slice it, **good nutrition is the secret to experiencing good health**.

Dr. Francis M. Pottenger, Jr., a medical doctor and researcher in the early 20th century, observed that heat processing destroys the nutritional content of food. Further, when fed to animals during the early stages of growth and development, inferior nutrition undermined the health of those animals.

In fact, consumption of cooked and processed food caused body malformations, arthritis, chronic diseases and also reduced reproductive capacity. By the third generation of his subject animals, they were too arthritic to crawl to the food set aside in their cages. Dr. Pottenger found that the situation could be reversed by feeding his cats the foods nature intended for them to eat, raw foods, but it took four generations to do it! (For the complete story, read ***Pottenger's Cats: A Study in Nutrition*** by Francis M. Pottenger, Jr., MD.)

This genetic decline is the opposite of the snowball effect; health gets weaker, not stronger, as it flows downhill. In other words, with each subsequent generation of people who are insufficiently nourished comes the weakening of the genetic pool.

As I do not consider myself to be a conspiracist, I would like to believe that all of this was inadvertent, and that's true to a large degree. But it doesn't end there. A closer look at history reveals a picture of both inadvertent *and* active suppression. For proof of this, I direct your attention to a prime example: Dr. Royal Lee, the founder of Standard Process vitamin company.

Dr. Lee was born in 1885. He was a dentist – as well as an inventor, a researcher, a scientist, a scholar, a statesman, a businessman and a philanthropist. As an inventor, he ultimately held some 100 patents, including the Lee electric governor, which enabled electric motors to be run at various speeds.

This technology was used in equipment as varied as radar, calculating machines, food mixers, flame cutters, fusion welders, drill presses, telephones and motion pictures. Dr. Lee's genius for the deciphering of working things was so universally admired that, in 1967, NASA called him to work out a means and method for recycling wastes into drinking water for astronauts.

But his first love was always health and nutrition. He produced his first vitamin product, Catalyn, in 1929. This foundational supplement would be the first of many raw food concentrates his Vitamin Products Company, now known as Standard Process, would formulate.

By 1941, Dr. Lee organized the Lee Foundation for Nutritional Research. As David Morris, DO, wrote in his article, *"Royal Lee, DDS: Father of Natural Vitamins,"* Dr. Lee's foundation became the world's largest clearinghouse for nutritional information for doctors, agriculturists and homemakers. By the way, he was paid $1 per year from both of these organizations during his lifetime. Not that Dr. Lee wasn't a firm believer in free enterprise, but nutrition and health improvement were his passions.

One startling discovery he highlighted was that, as a chemical complex, vitamins could be detected using refractive light. He used this discovery to show that synthetic vitamins (that is, those put together in a laboratory) could not function in the same way as those that occurred naturally in foods. The reason was simple: Although they may have the same chemical composition, natural and synthetic vitamins refract light oppositely.

An example of this principle is the comparison of dextrose (glucose) to levulose; both of these are forms of sugar. They have the same chemical composition, but dextrose (which is chemically derived from corn starch) has a right-handed twist and levulose (a monosaccharide found in sweet fruits and honey) has a left-handed twist. This is not their only difference: Dextrose contributes to the advance of diabetes while levulose does not. **Yes, the synthetic**

form causes disease while the natural form does not. And this single fact is why most of you, despite your taking supplements, do not experience improved health.

In fact, you may even be aggravating your condition.

We often see articles where claims for vitamin efficacy are tested only to disappoint. The biggest reason for this phenomenon is that synthetic vitamins don't work as nutritional support. If they work at all, it's in a pharmacological sense. In other words, they work **just like a drug**. They can even cause ill effects, as was proven many years ago in an animal study of vitamin E (D-alpha tocopheral) in which the poor unfortunate subjects became sterile. (So much for your synthetic vitamin E intake today.)

Now, this **should** be headline news!

Are you aware of this study? Did you catch it last night on CNN or even MSNBC? Are the paparazzi stalking the researchers with embarrassing questions? Is Oprah starting a support group for the animal victims? Will it ever make the cover of *People*?

Hardly… This is because negative information about the ill effects of synthetic vitamins can affect the monetary profits of scientists, researchers and, most of all, vitamin company owners, whose sources for raw materials, by the way, are often chemical companies like Monsanto. These people are used to recording their profits in the "$billions" column, not the "$millions" column. With that kind of political lobbying clout, no wonder such studies are buried and not buoyed.

But not Royal Lee. Dr. Lee was dedicated to the proposition that health was about revealing the relationship between the most powerful healing tool on the planet – the miraculous human body – and the nutritional factors that maintained healthy function. This view was, and still is, in direct opposition to the "germ theory" held by the self-proclaimed "gods of disease" (i.e., mainstream medical professionals) who were and are dead set on curing disease with poisons (i.e. pharmaceuticals). Dr. Lee would often say, and I'm paraphrasing, "What sense does it make to give poison to a person in order to treat conditions brought about by starvation?"

As you would imagine, this view put him at odds not only with the medical establishment but also with the towering triad of government, processed food and pharmaceutical/chemical industries.

Dr. Lee spent many years – and much of his wealth – defending his progressive positions. The federal government actively spent years trying to put him out of business. Along the way, it successfully suppressed literature that would have informed the public of many of his revelations. This was done under the guise of protecting the public's so-called "well-being." And who are the beneficiaries of this subterfuge? That's right: the pharmaceutical and food-processing industries.

You see, the late 19th to early 20th centuries produced competing notions about health and how to stay healthy; what the cause of disease was and how to live quality lives. There were physicians who subscribed to what I'm calling the Naturalist school, who felt first and foremost that nutrition played a large role in our health and ability to withstand disease.

Their unwritten motto was essentially: take care of the body and the body will take care of you. They emphasized supporting the body's innate healing abilities, which they felt would prevent disease before it got started – or at least correct functional illnesses.

Functional illnesses are those that, for example, affect the operation of an organ rather than the structure of an organ.

The other view focused on forces outside the body. The discovery of germs like bacteria and viruses were their calling cards. The "germ theory" of disease was their mantra. Louis Pasteur, hailed as the father of this theory, became known to all for, among other things, his process called pasteurization. He and his colleagues discounted that poor nutrition laid the groundwork for disease. Their focus was on pathology: Study the body during the disease process and identify the "bugs" present. Kill the bug and you'll destroy disease.

In my opinion, this is a lot like closing the barn door once the horse is outside. The first step should be to build a strong immune system, and for that you need whole food nutrition with all of its enzymes, vitamins, minerals and trace elements. Because of the quote attributed to him, "The terrain (body) is everything, the bacteria is nothing," there remains a swirling controversy based on whether or not Pasteur all but recanted "bugs" as the cause of disease. Whether this true or not we'll never know for sure.

However, despite competing theories regarding the cause of disease, the "germ theory" remains the dominant paradigm today.

The effect of the germ theory in Pasteur's day was to shift personal responsibility for maintaining health to the medical profession. This was aptly described **in the book by Arthur Baker,** *Awakening Our Self Healing Body:* **"With the germ theory of disease, no longer did we have to take responsibility for sickness caused by our own transgressions of the laws of health. Instead we blamed germs for invading the body. The germ theory effectively shifted personal responsibility for health and well-being onto the shoulders of the medical profession which supposedly knew how to kill off the offending germs. Our own health slipped from our control."**

But what about life-threatening infections? Well, there is no doubt that antibiotics have saved many an individual from certain death. Infection was a significant cause of death prior to this discovery. However, people in the know attribute a reduction in deaths due to infection largely to improvements in public sanitation (such as clean sources of water, proper sewage systems and disinfecting techniques like washing your hands) rather than to antibiotics. But to apply the lessons of acute life-saving care treatment to every illness is misguided and, frankly, unwise.

We can compare our bodies to a house, and the various organs and glands of our bodies to the appliances that keep a happy house running effectively. Keep your house in order and it will keep you warm and dry, right? But just as you wouldn't think of destroying your whole house because the water faucet leaks (you would just fix the faucet), so too you shouldn't apply antibiotics every time someone gets a runny nose (a leaky faucet).

Antibiotics kill off more than just the "bad bugs." They kill the "good bugs," too. Bugs, and there are trillions of them, are an integral part of our immune system, the very system that protects us from disease. And while there has been an increase in warnings against the overuse of antibiotics, many doctors continue to prescribe them for such things as the common flu.

The fact is that flu is a virus – and viruses do not respond to antibiotics. This haphazard practice not only undermines individual immune systems but, on a larger scale, has created a team of "super bugs" that are increasingly resistant to our drugs. In this case, the cure really is worse than the disease.

Thus the vicious cycle continues.

The contention of the Naturalists – and my own as well – is that more often than not functional illness has more to do with nutritional deficiencies and the lack of knowledge of the individual's true needs in the environment in which he or she operates. The answer? Correct a person's nutrition and provide tools to operate in the environment according to personal needs and many degenerative and functional illnesses will be resolved. These include chronic illnesses like fatigue, allergies, pain, high blood pressure, heart disease, arthritis and so many others.

The bottom line is that personal accountability is key to monitoring your own dietary intake. We need to stop treating doctors, vitamins and quick cure-all remedies as salvation and more like support. If proper nutrition is the secret to unlocking maximum health, then only we can hold the key.

Health Heist Handbook:

*The promise of good adult health is dependent on two key factors: **good genes** AND **good nutrition**.*
There's not much to do about the one, but you've certainly got control over the other!

Chapter 6

The Great Health Heist

So why did I title this book *The Great Health Heist*? Because, in no uncertain terms, your health has been stolen! And not by any hooded villain or armed robber, but by the very people you trust to give you sound medical advice.

That's right. Doctors, the food industry, the pharmaceutical industry and even the federal government are all complicit in perpetuating **the illusion that our food and drug supply is safe**. Further, they have replaced both common sense and science with the misplaced belief that health depends on some undiscovered silver bullet rather than with the underlying basics of **nutrition.**

Thanks to modern conveniences and on-the-go eating promoted by our fast-paced lifestyles – fast food, processed food, zapped food, frozen food, quick food, junk food and downright fake food – **we are starving and haven't the slightest clue.**

Moreover, good health does not just rely on good *post*-natal nutrition, but on *pre*-natal nutrition as well. I'm referring not only to your parents but also to their parents and their parents' parents. That's right: What your parents ate and were exposed to has a significant effect on **who you are** and **what type of health you may experience**.

The purposeful perpetrators of *The Great Health Heist* are getting away with more and more each day, and show no sign of being "arrested" anytime soon. For when it comes to power and greed, there appears to be no prisoners taken.

In the current health paradigm, the mistaken notion that disease is caused by germs predominates: not because of science, per se, but because of spreadsheets. It is simply more profitable for the medical and pharmacological community to kill germs than to create health.

Other forces of money and politics have skewed the world we now grapple with. Dr. Harvey Wiley (1844-1930) was the founder of the Pure Food and Drug Act, signed into law by Theodore Roosevelt in 1906. He was also the first director of the Bureau of Chemistry, now known as the United States Food and Drug Administration (FDA).

Dr. Wiley envisioned this governmental agency to be the protector of the public health, especially the food supply. The Pure Food and Drug Act prohibited the addition of any ingredients that would substitute for the food, conceal damage, pose a health hazard or constitute a filthy or decomposed substance.

He challenged the grain industry for bleaching flour. This process required the addition of chlorine dioxide, which was found to react with wheat proteins, creating a diabetes-causing contaminant alloxan. He took the case all the way to the Supreme Court of the United States, and won. Unfortunately, while the ruling was a victory for a safer food supply, it went unheeded and unenforced.

To add insult to injury, Dr. Wiley was removed from the agency he created in favor of Dr. Elmer M. Nelson, a former executive of the Pillsbury Foods Company, purveyors of processed grains. Recall the Pillsbury Doughboy? (Although the Doughboy icon wasn't created by the ad agency Leo Burnett Worldwide of Chicago until the 1970s.)

Any questions?

The Great Health Heist begins.

If you're looking for one of the original deceivers who set the stage for *The Great Health Heist*, you've just found him: Elmer M. Nelson. This man perpetuated the pivotal argument used even today by naysayers that nutrition has very little connection with resistance to disease. He set the tone for government policy by stating, "It is wholly unscientific to state that a well-fed body is more able to resist disease than a less well-fed body. My overall opinion is that there hasn't been enough experimentation to prove dietary deficiencies make one more susceptible to disease." (*Washington Post*; October 26, 1949.)

Of course today, nearly 60 years later, we know differently! Right? NOT!! Knowledge and action are two very different things. My parents would always say, "Actions speak louder than words." I readily admit that there are movements afoot to shine the spotlight on the importance of nutrition – and there are plenty of nutritionists about. But, to this day, the majority of medical schools spend only **a few hours** educating doctors about nutrition!

And when vitamins were discovered and found to be present in food as well as to be essential to fostering good health, instead of emphasizing the consumption of whole foods, the soon-to-be pharmaceutical industrial complex set about trying to identify single active ingredients that could be synthesized, reproduced cheaply in factories and, most importantly, patented.

Food conglomerates set about (1) processing foods to taste good and (2) enriching them to overcome the alteration of their real food value. Despite their products' obvious shortcomings, the food industry trumpets their nutritional benefits. By **spraying synthetic vitamins on their goods** – vitamins that don't work, by the way – somewhere in the process, **they are allowed to claim "high vitamin content."** Moreover, they often claim preventative health benefits using sound bites like "heart healthy" and "enriched."

As a nation, we respond in a Pavlovian manner; salivating at the mere thought of eating quickly – and healthily – without ever having to fire up a stove or crack open an egg. It's only human nature. Hear these things often enough and people begin to believe it. Conspiring right along with these folks is the federal government in its proclamation that all is well – and that all subsequent drugs and chemicals used both in suppressing symptoms and in food production are safe.

The actors are in place; the strategy is clear. Thus the stage has been set for *The Great Health Heist*. Yes, that's right. When The Powers That Be convince us they have "our well-being" in mind, eventually most of us come to believe it. After all, it's "heart healthy," right? They have effectively created a diversion and, as a result, robbed us of our power – and our health.

And while these events are taking place, they are also actively trying to eliminate safe, natural and effective means of treating so many functional illnesses. These tools lay scattered and hidden, only to be resurrected by healthcare practitioners and individuals like you and me, who could not find answers to their illnesses.

We have been (and continue to be) made to suffer not only with our illnesses, but also with the side effects of drugs. We are, as Dr. Strand so aptly concludes in **Death by Prescription**, the "grand clinical trial for thousands of poisonous drugs." Belittled for questioning the wisdom of their use and helpless because we feel we don't have the expertise to find an alternative, we are at the mercy of doctors and the healthcare system that feeds them.

All of us know that medical care costs $20-25, or whatever your particular co-pay might be. But co-pays approximate nowhere near the real costs of healthcare. The pact that insurance companies made back in the mid-20th century with the American Medical Association (AMA), which allowed doctors to charge whatever they wanted for their services, is failing.

Insurance companies now feel the pressure and are making every effort to pass on the costs to us in the form of higher premiums while reducing reimbursements to physicians. And everyone is feeling the pinch: groups, companies, doctors, patients and the federal and state governments. Our healthcare system ranks 37th out of all industrialized nations. $6,711 is spent on every man, woman and child in this country while our overall health continues to erode.

This is the predicament we find ourselves in.

This is the great health heist!

Dr. Royal Lee, founder of Standard Process whole-food nutritional products, spoke prescient words when he said:

"We have drifted into this deplorable position of national malnutrition quite inadvertently. It is the result of scientific research with the objective of finding the best ways to create foods that are non-perishable, that can be made by mass production methods in

central factories, and distributed so cheaply that they can sweep all local competition from the market...Then, after there develops a suspicion that these 'foods' are inadequate to support life, modern advertising steps in to propagandize the people into believing that there is nothing wrong with them, that they are products of scientific research intended to afford a food that is the last word in nutritive value and the confused public is totally unable to arrive at any conclusion of fact, and continues to blindly buy the rubbish that is killing them years ahead of their time."

~ Dr. Royal Lee; June 1943

1943? Sounds like it could have been said last year, last month; sounds like it could have been said yesterday! While focusing on the germs, the group in power ignored the simple but powerful tool of *nutrition*.

In their zeal to make money, food companies ignore the well-being of their customers by producing food products that are inferior and cause functional illness. Pharmaceutical companies know that a patent for a product is worth more money than a whole food could ever be. So, producing drug products that are able to suppress symptoms appear to "cure" the disease.

Once again here is what Dr. Lee said:

"One of the biggest tragedies of human civilization is the precedence of chemical therapy over nutrition. It's a substitution of artificial therapy over natural, of poisons over food, in which we are feeding people poison in trying to correct the reactions of starvation."

~ Dr. Royal Lee; January 12, 1951

And, finally, the federal government (in the form of the FDA), which is supposed to provide safety and protection from health threats such as harmful medications, now fast tracks drugs **without thorough testing**. Further, more than half of the money for that testing comes from the pharmaceutical industry itself.

Kind of like the fox guarding the hen house again, wouldn't you agree?

What makes the safety issue even worse is that the whole system depends upon voluntary reporting of problems with drugs.

That's right. Are the drug companies going to blow the whistle on themselves after spending hundreds of millions of dollars producing and advertising their product? I don't think so!

Thus, the greatest heist, our health, was set in motion. It all began quite inadvertently in the late 19th to early 20th centuries. The usual suspects formed an alliance and chose their weapons in the form of greed, power and deception.

But we are victims no more!

They stole our health – now we must take it back!

Health Heist Handbook:

*It is simply more profitable for the medical and pharmacological community to **kill germs** rather than **foster health**.*

Part 2

Nutrition Response Testing^{SM}

Chapter 7

What is Nutrition Response Testing?

What is science?

What is magic?

Are the two indistinguishable?

In *Profiles of the Future*, Arthur C. Clarke spoke to the "Limits of the Possible" when he wrote, "Any sufficiently advanced technology is indistinguishable from magic."

For those of you who don't know, Arthur C. Clarke was a prolific science fiction writer as well as an inventor. He was largely responsible for conceiving the satellite system currently revolving around Earth, allowing for the cell-phone communication and GPS tracking that we enjoy today. In addition, he was nominated for an Academy Award for best screenplay when he collaborated with the director Stanley Kubrick on *2001: A Space Odyssey*.

Clarke made a brilliant point in likening science to magic; one often feels, or at least looks, like the other. Think back to the wonderful medical discoveries throughout the ages and you'll realize that public reaction was often similar to that of the Salem residents and their "witch trials."

We've all seen illustrations of leeches being used in colonial times to bleed victims and rid them of their various ailments. How magical must surgery have seemed when it was first introduced to the world?

And what must the locals have thought when, in the late 1790s, Edward Jenner purposefully injected a young boy with the pus from a cowpox sore to prevent infection from smallpox? While the results were indeed magical, the name was quite real: vaccination. Today we take vaccines for granted, forgetting that over 200 years ago the feat was likened to heresy although currently, controversy swirls over the safety of vaccinations.

For doubters, science is often seen as **magic**. For the curious, science is always revered as **knowledge**. That's because the very word "science" comes from the Latin word *scire,* meaning "to know." We commonly understand science to mean knowledge, or a system of knowledge, covering general truths or the operation of general laws, especially as obtained and tested through the scientific method.

Although the basis for the Scientific Method is attributed to Robert Grosseteste, an English bishop who lived in the 12th century, Francis Bacon, a 17th century English philosopher, is credited with popularizing what is known today as the inductive scientific method. His methodology, a methodical observation of facts as a means of studying and interpreting natural phenomenon, remains the viable framework for scientific investigation today. His reformulation was his reaction to the all too fanciful guessing and to the mere citing of existing authorities of the time. Bacon's method is commonly referred to as the empirical method. Empirical means originating in or based upon observation or experience.

Because Bacon's method was a reaction to the system in place at the time, it was criticized for disregarding the theory and systems in place. Think where we would be today if people did not challenge the theories and systems currently in place. And you don't have to be a scientist to challenge the status quo.

Dr. Martin Luther King, Jr., challenged the status quo. His challenge led to the Civil Rights Movement and more equality among the races.

Susan B. Anthony challenged the status quo. Her challenge led to the Suffrage Movement and more equal rights for women.

You might counter that there is still a disparity among races, not to mention between the sexes, but how much *more* of a disparity might there be without these bold thinkers, doers and, yes, social scientists?

Health, like equality, politics or even science, is not the quest for an unattainable perfection, but the journey toward the best your body, mind and spirit can be. Health is an ongoing process reliant on a variety of factors, including (1) your own motivation to succeed; (2) tools like whole food concentrates and herbs that work; (3) live, fresh, unadulterated foods; (4) knowledge that brings results; (5) a dogged determination and persistence and, above all, (6) knowing that there really is **HOPE**.

After all, progress is best exemplified by the fact that theories and systems are leapfrogged based on subsequent discoveries. These discoveries are often based on empirical observation.

Nutrition Response Testing is an empirically based technology that is systematic, repeatable and, most importantly, predictably effective.

RESULTS! What else do you need?

Where Did It Originate?

Nutrition Response Testing was composed and refined by Freddie Ulan, D.C., C.C.N., and Lester Bryman, D.C., C.D.N. It is based on decades of successful clinical outcomes helping sick people restore their health naturally – without drugs, without surgery, non-invasively and often relatively rapidly.

Nutrition Response Testing combines knowledge of the autonomic nervous system (ANS), the body's system that controls all vital functions including metabolism (the chemical processes that occur in your body to maintain life) and repair, with the breakthroughs in applied and clinical kinesiology developed in the early 1960s. Nutrition Response Testing utilizes the most workable advancements and refinements in the field, including those of several notable medical researchers.

In this system, we do not "diagnose" or "treat" diseases. Instead, we use revolutionary tools that allow the trained practitioner to obtain a highly dependable assessment of a patient's current health status.

Combined with an understanding of anatomy, physiology, neurology, kinesiology and biochemistry, the assessment allows the trained practitioner to actually identify and correct the underlying causes of "dis-ease" rather than simply suppress symptoms.

What is Nutrition Response Testing?

Nutrition Response Testing is a technology that obtains critical information about bodily function from the autonomic nervous system (ANS). Autonomic refers to something that occurs involuntarily. Bodily functions like eye blinking, heart and breathing rates, digestive metabolism, immune response, hormone regulation and so forth are regulated by the ANS. There are two controls to the ANS:

1. **Sympathetic**
2. **Parasympathetic**

Think of them as our body's accelerator (sympathetic control) and brake (parasympathetic control) – our "go" pedal and "whoa" pedal. When our bodies are healthy and in balance, these systems function properly and are in tune with one another; the sympathetic dominates when we are active, the parasympathetic when we are resting.

These regulators are responsible for healthy functioning, including our ability to heal. It is when there is an imbalance, blockage or interference that we experience symptoms such as allergies, acid reflux, high blood pressure, chronic pain, headaches and the like. Think of these symptoms as "check engine lights" or "alarm bells." These imbalances can be corrected safely, naturally and effectively by accessing the ANS.

The 3-P Method and the 5 Stressors

The 3-P Method refers to the fact that the Nutrition Response Testing technique is **Painless**, **Powerful** and **Personalized**. This empirically proven technique allows us to accurately determine what stands in the way between you and better health. In fact, Dr. Ulan's discovery of the barriers to healing he called **stressors** "...opened the door to the most effective, most economical, easiest-to-comply-with, lowest-pill-count program ever." And that, says Dr. Ulan, "is the key secret to our success."

When undergoing Nutrition Response Testing you will be tested for these five common stressors:

1. **Scars**
2. **Food sensitivities**
3. **Immune challenges**
4. **Chemical challenges**
5. **Metal challenges**

These stressors can and will prevent your body from healing. Many of you have experienced this already without perhaps realizing it. Have you ever failed to respond to perfectly good treatment? Have you ever experienced the opposite result to perfectly good treatment? Has your condition "plateaued" or gotten better and then worse? If so, these are all indications that your body isn't fully open to healing. Nutrition Response Testing allows the practitioner to test you using the "stressors" to reveal and then remove these barriers.

Next, specific organ reflexes are tested (such as liver, heart and bowel) as well as glandular reflexes (like prostate, thyroid and adrenals). Then the priority reflex is determined. This step is critical to Nutrition Response Testing because pinpointing the priority results in having to take fewer supplements, achieving a lowered pill count and a phenomenon I call "whole body healing." Have you ever just gotten temporary relief or relief of some but not all of your symptoms? If so, then you haven't achieved whole body healing.

Based on this determination, we will recommend specific whole-food supplements and/or herbs as well as dietary and lifestyle changes. This is all done painlessly, with the practitioner lightly pressing on different acupuncture points or reflex locations on the body associated with specific organs or glands, while simultaneously checking a strong muscle group.

The result is a **personalized health improvement program** that addresses your own body's imbalances and corrects its operation. Our goals are two-fold: **achieving good health** and **feeling good again** – safely, naturally and effectively. You are bound to get results as long as you follow your personalized program.

Accessing the Autonomic Nervous System (ANS)

We use a standardized form of applied kinesiology, commonly known as muscle testing. In the hands of thoroughly trained health professionals, this highly effective method of evaluation gives the practitioner essential information about your body's requirements for a return to health. Book learning and clinical experience, which are the sum total of theoretical and educated knowledge, can clearly help us get close to what may be required to pinpoint the solution to your health concerns. But what separates Nutrition Response Testing from most other treatment strategies is the critical information obtained from the body itself or, as we say, **accessing the body's innate intelligence in order to find the precise answers to your health concerns.**

Who Can Benefit from Our Nutritional Healing Program?

Men!

Women!

Children!

Take your pick. Anyone who wants to improve their health – or maintain the good health they currently enjoy. Anyone who wants to lose weight naturally and effectively without drugs or "miracle diets." Anyone who wants to boost their energy level, curb their sugar or carbohydrate cravings or take less medication. In other words, anyone who seriously wants to address his or her own body's "dis-ease!"

What Conditions Can It Address?

A better question might be, "What *can't* Nutrition Response Testing address?" Here is just a partial list of conditions we address and conquer on a daily basis at my clinic:

- Weight control
- Fatigue
- Stress

- Depression
- Acid reflux
- ADHD

- Allergies
- Arthritis
- Asthma
- Bloating
- High blood pressure
- Candida
- High cholesterol
- Chronic pain
- Colds and flu
- Constipation
- Diarrhea
- Food sensitivities
- Headaches and migraines
- Heart conditions
- IBS/IBD
- Infertility
- Menopause and PMS
- Multiple sclerosis
- Osteoporosis
- Skin/hair/nail issues
- Tremors
- And many others

What Improvements Will I Notice on My Program?

Simply put, you'll get better! Many patients see dramatic changes in a few short weeks. But Rome wasn't built in a day and, for most of you, your health didn't fall apart in a day either.

Western medicine, led on by the pharmaceutical giants (with plenty of help from the media), has capitalized on your desire for instantaneous relief even though it leads to more complications down the road. They offer toxic poisons in the form of drugs to treat the symptoms of starvation.

Well, you now have a **safe, natural and effective option**. But it must be emphasized that it may take a period of months for you to witness your health's transformation. After all, a garden doesn't come to fruition overnight and our bodies are compensating for a lot of previous abuse!

What is the Nutrition Response Program?

The Nutrition Response Program is an individualized health improvement program designed to restore normal bodily function. The reason we succeed where others have failed is because we access the body's innate intelligence and combine it with our educated intelligence.

Testing for Heart Rate Variability (HRV)

Heart Rate Variability, or HRV, is a fully automatic, noninvasive, computer-based system designed to assess physical fitness and the functional balance of the automatic nervous system (ANS). It is the autonomic nervous system that acupuncture, homeopathy and chiropractic rely on to accomplish changes in bodily function.

Clinical tests conducted at Columbia University Medical Center have confirmed the HRV testing system to be over 95% accurate in its assessment when compared to industry standards. It accurately determines your heart's ability to respond to daily stress. Lastly, it provides a numerical score and graph that reports how healthy you are.

We Found the Answer – Now You Can, Too!

This section of the book is full of brief testimonials, stories from people who have chosen or were forced to seek alternatives to their personal and inadvertent health tragedies. You've already read my story. Now read about others just like me who found the science – the magic – of good health!

My patients and I were not happy with our predicament. We made a change. We found hope and an effective solution by taking back our health. We recognized that we were accomplices to those who would steal our health from us; that the heist, at least in part, reflected our own reluctance to act. You can act, too. You are not a victim unless you accept that role.

You must act!

Please read on.

The science – the magic – of healing awaits!

Health Heist Handbook:

Health, like equality, politics or even science, is not the quest for perfection, but only the journey toward the best your body, mind and spirit can be.

Chapter 8

Weight Loss and Diabetes

I struggled with whether or not to start the "Symptoms and Ailments" section of this book with the subject of weight loss. On one hand, it is one of the most persistent and popular complaints mentioned by my patients. On the other hand, I hesitate to become part of the problem. By this I mean that I don't want to imply, by placing this chapter front and center, that weight loss is more important than, say, symptoms of painful conditions or even allergies.

Please understand that *all* of the maladies you'll be reading about, as well as the patient testimonials, are equally important. To whom? To you, the person suffering from them. In fact, **no** pain is more important than the one you are suffering from **at this very moment**. Be it arthritis, post-surgical pain or simply persistent heartburn, physical suffering can become all-consuming. Pain grinds us down and shuts us off from the people we love, from what we do, and from how much we enjoy life.

So I'll begin this section with a quick caveat: Weight loss can be important, but in no way is Nutrition Response Testing a diet or weight-loss program. It just so happens that when you put Nutrition Response Testing and your personalized health improvement program to work your body immediately starts returning to that lovely state of balance, including restoring its power to heal.

As a result, patients first experience weight loss because of the release of accumulated toxic waste products trapped in your body's individual cells. Often weight in the form of fat continues to fall off because of dietary modifications and subtle metabolic changes. Overall, **balance is restored along with a strategy not only to get healthy but also to stay healthy**.

The bottom line – you'll feel better and look better.

Weight-loss programs abound, from those that sell prepared foods like NutriSystem to those that don't, like Jenny Craig and L.A. Weight Loss. Plentiful, too, are fad diets like Atkins, South Beach and Blood Type. There are almost as many approaches to weight loss as there are diets. So how do you decide? Where do you begin?

The key to losing weight is identifying specific individualized factors we call "hold ups." It's true that most everyone who reduces his or her caloric intake will lose weight. But once on your program of choice, did you fail to lose weight? Did you lose some weight and then stop or plateau? After you lost weight, did you feel healthier? Were you more energetic and free of symptoms? Were you able to maintain the weight-loss over time? Did you maintain your newly found health? Are you still looking for answers to any of these questions? If so, then you're definitely ready to identify your "hold ups" – your hidden health problems.

Beth, a 40-year-old single mom with two teenage children, had always been dedicated to her health and that of her family. Whenever faced with health concerns, she always chose alternative approaches. But she suffered with almost constant digestive problems, chronic mouth soreness, difficult menstrual cycles (linked to uterine fibroids so plentiful that doctors insisted she have a hysterectomy to avoid cancer) and excess weight. She was devoted to a vegetarian lifestyle that included the consumption of soy and dairy products.

After her evaluation using Nutrition Response Testing, soy along with dairy were identified as foods she was sensitive to. Within one week of eliminating them from her diet, Beth's digestive complaints and mouth soreness disappeared. Her fibroids ultimately vanished, along with her difficult menstrual cycles, and she avoided a hysterectomy.

Following years of trying to lose weight, within two weeks she lost over 10 pounds. All told, she has lost over 80 pounds. The process has taken three years, with several periods of rest or what are often referred to as "plateaus." Today, her hair, skin and nails are vibrant and her health remains elevated as she rarely finds herself prone to colds.

But don't take Beth's word for it. This chapter is loaded with testimonials from people just like her who've discovered Nutrition Response Testing. They've embraced their personalized health improvement program as a healthy, safe and proven alternative to those fad diets that, let's face it, rarely work.

These folks found the answer to the question you've been asking for a long time – why haven't those fad diets worked for me? More fundamentally, how do I decide which one to choose in the first place?

Take Virginia, who wrote, *"I thought I was very healthy. I worked long hours, slept well and took too little time off, but I had a dry cough that was embarrassing, I craved sweets and wanted to lose weight. I squeezed into Curves once a day for one month and managed to lose five pounds. [But my symptoms remained]. [After being evaluated using Nutrition Response Testing and being on my program], my cough disappeared unless I ate foods I was supposed to avoid. What's more, I've lost 10 pounds and my sugar cravings AND I've had compliments about my [new] appearance."*

I hear this refrain from many patients. It seems as if the ongoing battle to lose weight has taken over their lives. Finding a process that helps them control their weight really helps them feel rejuvenated and, more importantly, restores their hope for a better quality of life.

As part of this rejuvenation we experience less brain fog, more emotional stability and **more energy**. I liken weight loss to unpacking a heavy backpack during a long, arduous hike. The more weight we carry, the harder it is to climb, jog, walk or sprint. As we shed pounds, our body's "backpack" gets lighter and our movements easier. More energy is a very natural and welcome result.

The problem with most weight-loss programs, however, is that they don't result in whole-body wellness; their sole target is weight loss and the rest is optional. As a result, many people on these shortsighted programs get only half-hearted results – or none at all. The point is they continue to experience some chronic symptoms and they are often the victims of the dreaded dieter's plateau.

"AD" hit the dieter's plateau – and hard. *"Before the [Nutrition Response Testing] program,"* he explained, *"I had lost about 10 pounds following a low carbohydrate diet. My weight stayed the same for at least a year. When I started seeing Paul for Nutrition Response Testing, I had a number of symptoms I wanted to address and weight was one of them. Since I have been tested, I have lost 15 pounds. It was difficult at first to figure out what foods to eat, but a few weeks into the program it got easier and easier. I like this plan because I don't have to count calories, fat grams, or carbohydrates. I simply don't eat the four foods I tested negative for. Not only have I lost weight, but also I feel better emotionally as well. I react to crisis and sadness in my life much better now."*

Plateaus are a common challenge with many weight-loss programs. Here is another similar story with an equally happy ending. "RR" suffered from a stubborn weight-loss plateau and fatigue, a standard combination that in my profession seems to go together like burgers and fries.

"My weight loss had plateaued despite being on a low carb diet," explains "RR." *"My energy was down. I had to drink coffee to*

make it through the day. My weight loss resumed three days after starting the [Nutrition Response Testing] program. Now I have increased, dependable energy. I was able to stop drinking coffee...."

"RR" quickly discovered – in three days, no less – the causal relationship between overcoming a weight-loss plateau and experiencing more energy. This causal relationship is one enjoyed by many of my patients. Take "BW" for instance.

"[After Nutrition Response Testing] my energy level is much higher than it has been for a long time now. I have lost 8-10 pounds without doing anything different other than changing my diet and taking the supplements."

All of these enthusiastic patients learned that weight loss is more than just about fitting back into those jeans you wore last year or buying a whole new wardrobe in a smaller size. They were touched by whole body wellness.

Weight loss is a function of weight management. But more importantly, that management must be based on a personalized health improvement program designed to achieve whole body wellness. Much like we need to get off the pharmaceutical bandwagon and quit believing the hype about "a pill for every ill," so, too, do we need to quit focusing on weight loss alone as the panacea to whole body wellness.

We must quit believing that "starvation leads to salvation!"

Health Heist Handbook:

Be it arthritis, post-surgical pain or simply persistent heartburn, pain can become all-consuming; it grinds us down, shutting us off from those we love, what we do and even how much we enjoy life.

Diabetes

Over 20 million people are type-2 diabetics, with another 54 million ready to join their ranks as pre-diabetics. The scary part is that over half the pre-diabetics don't even know they are in danger.

In a June 19, 2007 article, Reuters reported that one out of every eight U.S. federal health care dollars is spent treating people with diabetes. The study, based on federal spending data from 2005, found that it cost $79.7 billion more to treat people with diabetes than those without. As of 2002, over $132 billion was spent treating diabetes and all it's complications. This last figure will surely rise.

Sales of medicines to treat diabetes are projected to soar 60-68 percent by 2009 from 2006 levels. In 2005, total drug sales reached almost $10 billion. And over the next 30 years, diabetes is expected to claim the lives of 62 million Americans.

What exactly *is* diabetes? According to the American Diabetes Association (ADA), *"Diabetes is a disease in which the body does not produce or properly use insulin. Insulin is a hormone that is needed to convert sugar, starches and other food into energy needed for daily life. The cause of diabetes continues to be a mystery, although both genetics and environmental factors such as obesity and lack of exercise appear to play roles."*

Unfortunately, the ADA appears to be one of the main reasons diabetics remain diabetic, especially those diagnosed with type 2 symptoms. For one thing, despite the 2005 revision of the government's food pyramid both versions recommend consuming whole grains. This is not necessarily a bad thing but in the case of a diabetic, the ADA's failure to warn off such consumption is concerning. This is because grains, like sugar and other concentrated sweeteners, are high-glycemic foods and cause a spike in insulin production, simply adding to a diabetic's insulin resistance. And I am here to tell you: **Any diabetic who continues to eat grains (things like bread, pasta, tortillas and Chinese take-out rice), while thinking it is okay, is simply in denial. Such a person is misinformed and doing him or herself great harm!** For another, Western medicine and the ADA subscribe to the notion that diabetes is a disease of blood sugar. But high blood sugar is the symptom of diabetes, not the cause. Current research reveals that diabetes is actually a disease of hormone signaling. Normal hormone signaling, or control, depends on a "happy" endocrine system. Normalize the endocrine system and you've got the solution.

Comprised of the glands (pituitary, pineal, thyroid, thymus, pancreas, which is a digestive organ as well, ovaries/testis and adrenals) and the hormones they produce, the endocrine system regulates most of the body's organs, cells and their functions. Acting as a kind of "command central," the endocrine system helps regulate mood, metabolism, development and growth, tissue function and reproduction.

Moreover, the proper functioning of the endocrine system, especially as it relates to the pancreas (the insulin-producing gland), depends on a fully functional autonomic nervous system (autonomic meaning self-regulating or regulating without your willful control); both of these systems must be unhindered and properly nourished to maintain normal operation. If you are pre-diabetic or a confirmed diabetic, herein lies the rub.

If you don't find the hidden health problems hindering your endocrine and/or autonomic nervous systems and focus only on managing blood sugar, then you will remain a diabetic for life. Well, now you have a choice! Why fight your pains and ills with one hand tied behind your back?

So how do we restore proper operation to your endocrine system? Answer: by using Nutrition Response Testing to find the missing piece, which is your body's hidden health problem. And for heaven's sake, stop eating grains and sugar. When you make a commitment to follow your new personalized health improvement program to the letter, you will have no more blood sugar problems.

"Bill," a middle-aged man in otherwise good health, had recently been given bad news. His blood sugars were climbing. He was put on an oral drug, Metformin, and told to watch his diet. Fortunately for Bill, the drugs were not working well. He noticed that the symptoms he suffered (fatigue, brain fog and migrating body pains) just got worse. After a good deal of soul searching, he reached a crossroads. He decided to pursue alternative methods to handle his blood sugar problems and responded to my radio program, "Health Matters," in Portland, Oregon.

After undergoing an evaluation at my clinic, Bill got his individualized health improvement program and started following it. Within two weeks, his blood sugars dropped. His brain was clear and he found his energy returning to a less painful body. As of this writing, his blood sugars are normal without any medication.

Health Heist Handbook:

Over the next 30 years, diabetes is expected to claim the lives of 62 million Americans.

Chapter 9

Fatigue, Insomnia and General Malaise

Often I see patients who can't pinpoint their ills, syndromes or special conditions. There is no simple box for them to check or blank for them to fill in on the intake form where you record what ails you. They, like so many Americans, suffer from fatigue, poor sleep (often labeled insomnia) and what I call a "general sense of malaise" that is both insidious and disastrous.

Many of these patients feel guilty about complaining because, really, they have no specific complaint. They can't put a label on how they feel, so they say nothing. And gradually this fatigue, insomnia and general malaise gets worse. They wake up morning after morning, feeling ten to twenty years older, and always behind the eight ball. They can't understand why they just don't feel good and why other people seem so happy, joyful, lively and full of zest.

They don't know **what's wrong**; they just know **something's wrong**.

Americans like to label things. We like definitions, buzz words, catchphrases and, in particular, diagnoses that suit us exactly. High cholesterol, overactive bladder, arthritis, hypertension, even stress are all conditions easily identified, quickly labeled and conveniently "suppressed" or "managed", not cured, mind you. These conditions are commonly managed using toxic prescription drugs, all of which have harmful side effects.

But what about symptoms that aren't neatly categorized on the intake forms you fill out at your healthcare practitioner's office? What if there's not enough space on the little blank marked "Other" for you to explain why you just don't feel right?

How do we label that? How do we treat it? How do we cure it? Unfortunately, and more often than we'd like to realize, many such people are labeled with depression and walk out of their doctor's offices with antidepressant medications like Prozac or Zoloft – more drugs with harmful side effects.

In this chapter I discuss three conditions common to this generally unpleasant feeling of "something's wrong with me; I just don't know what" condition and provide a drug-free alternative:

- **Fatigue Versus Chronic Fatigue**
- **Fatigue and Insomnia**
- **Adrenal Exhaustion or Thyroid Fatigue**

Health Heist Handbook:

*They don't know **what's wrong;***

*they just know **something's wrong**.*

Fatigue Versus Chronic Fatigue

What is the difference between fatigue and chronic fatigue? Where is the threshold between just plain feeling tired and just plain "sick and tired" of feeling tired? How do you know when your fatigue turns chronic? Or when it is no longer chronic?

The least scientific explanation I can give for the difference between fatigue and chronic fatigue is that it rarely matters to the person who is just plain tired. It just so happens that the most scientific explanation I can give for the difference between fatigue and chronic fatigue is that it rarely matters to the person who is just plain tired!

I'm not being flip; this is really how my patients feel about fatigue. Some come in right away because they've felt tired for a few days. Others wait until they've felt fatigued for months, sometimes even years, before they are tempted to consider the fact that their fatigue might be chronic.

The folks at MedicineNet.com determine **fatigue** to be "a condition characterized by a lessened capacity for work and reduced efficiency of accomplishment, usually accompanied by a feeling of weariness and tiredness." Sounds about right.

MedicineNet.com defines **chronic fatigue** as "a debilitating and complex disorder characterized by profound fatigue of six months or longer duration that is not improved by bed rest and that may be worsened by physical or mental activity."

Clearly, both definitions point to quantifiable and quite justifiable symptoms. Yet often there remains no specific laboratory test, or such tests fail to reveal anything obvious **or** reveal something that turns out to be the effect and not the root cause. The Centers for Disease Control, or CDC, insist that "as many as 500,000 Americans suffer from some type of chronic fatigue." I know this figure should be much higher because, in addition to the various specific maladies my patients report, fatigue and chronic fatigue are often co-symptoms.

"DM" came to me suffering from fatigue along with some other common symptoms I see quite often. Happily his story ended well. *"I didn't have the energy to do much, even with only working part time,"* he had complained. *"I usually felt worn out. Now [after Nutrition Response Testing], I feel more alert and positive. I wake up feeling more awake. I don't feel worn out even after exercising."*

In contrast, "FB" had symptoms that were slightly more aggravating. *"I was a basket case, tired, felt lousy and had no energy,"* she complained. *"I would have to push myself to do something. Now [after Nutrition Response Testing] I have more energy and get-up-and-go. It is not a struggle to do things."*

For "DM" and "FB," their complaints were generally fatigue-related. My next two patients weren't so lucky, and each suffered with chronic fatigue in their own unique way.

"LH" was diagnosed with chronic fatigue because of the duration and severity of his symptoms. Like many sufferers of this ailment, he had a combination of symptoms that went hand-in-hand with chronic fatigue. He explains: *"I was always tired, caught many colds that would last for weeks, had knee pain, low energy, and felt run down. Now [with Nutrition Response Testing], my energy is solid. I am able to hike for six to eight miles without the use of hiking poles. I haven't had any more colds or knee pain, and am sleeping well. I am feeling very healthy and strong."*

These symptoms were more severe than some sufferers of chronic fatigue, and less severe than others who fall victim to this insidious ailment. Take "MS," for instance. Like many who suffer from chronic fatigue, she found herself being misdiagnosed, again and again, by the established medical community. These are her words:

"I was experiencing extreme pain; I felt sick, weak, and could not eat or hold down any food. I went from doctor to doctor for 10 years trying to find out what or why my body was feeling the way it was. I went through multiple tests without finding a solution. I was told I would have to live like this, but this wasn't living. I felt like I was slowly dying. My weight had gone down to 100 pounds.

"I have been coming to see Paul Rosen for three months now. I have more strength, am able to eat some foods, and my weight is up to 117 pounds. I go out in public more and I'm not sick or in pain

like I was [after being on my Nutrition Response Testing program]. I feel stronger than I have in 10 years and feel like I'm actually going to make it back out into life again. I still have a long way to go, but this is all worth it."

Her problems may sound extreme, but symptoms like those experienced by "MS" are more common than you think. If they sound familiar, don't wait as long as she did – seek help now.

So what if you can't pinpoint your symptoms or put a name to what you are feeling? You know when your body is out of whack or isn't feeling right. And let me remind you about something: Don't ever be embarrassed about what a doctor or healthcare practitioner might think. They are just people with problems like yours and they are there to help.

If you are unhappy with the results of a particular treatment program, speak up and say so. Don't be passive. Be aggressive in the pursuit of better health – if, in fact, you are really willing to get down to work. Suspend your judgment and don't be afraid to pursue non-traditional methods. Demand that someone listen. Be persistent.

Better health, after all, can be yours – but you have to want it. I am here to tell you not to settle for the status quo while there is hope out there available to you. Don't be a victim of your current physical state. Overcome your fear and suspend your judgment. Now, there is an alternative.

Get evaluated using Nutrition Response Testing. It's painless. It's non-invasive. It will provide a personalized program with powerful results. Are you ready, as my spiritual teacher reminds us, to be the hero of your own life? What are you waiting for?

Health Heist Handbook:

The least scientific explanation I can give for the difference between fatigue and chronic fatigue is that it rarely matters to the person who is just plain tired.

Fatigue and Insomnia

Few maladies are as frustrating as the battle between fatigue and insomnia. This "circle of strife" feeds upon itself daily, making it harder to treat and more frustrating by degrees. Sleep becomes like the pot of gold at the end of a rainbow that is always just out of reach. As a result, it takes on an almost mythical presence; it consumes us and makes obtaining the sleep we need so badly even harder.

If you have ever suffered from insomnia, you know that it can be a horrific experience. Like a snowball getting bigger and bigger as it rolls downhill, the effects of insomnia combine throughout the days, the weeks, and even the months to create dozens of offshoot symptoms that make life miserable. Some of these include irritability, anxiety, diminishing physical performance and, not surprisingly, **fatigue**.

"EW" experienced this dreadful combination of insomnia plus fatigue recently and was kind enough to share his success story with us:

"I was tired through the day and had difficulty sleeping [insomnia]. I was concerned with my excess weight and not getting the results I was hoping for from cutting calories and exercise. [Following my Nutrition Response Testing evaluation], I am learning what types of food I should be eating and can tell now when I have eaten something I shouldn't have. I sleep soundly at night and

have a lot more energy throughout the day. In fact, I am working 50 to 60 hours a week and I have been able to stay energized throughout the long weeks. Everyone around me is constantly wondering how I have the energy to work these long hours and many of these people complain of their own lack of energy. Guess what? I am starting to refer my family and friends [to your clinic]!"

"LS" expressed the same type of frustration and ennui when she wrote me saying, *"I felt like I needed to do something different. I didn't know what, but I needed to do something."*

"LS" was fortunate that she had caring friends in the know. She explains:

"When I came to visit, my son, my daughter-in-law and my daughter Cindy convinced me to [be evaluated using Nutrition Response Testing]. I lacked the energy I had before three surgeries on my knee and a staph infection. I found I truly needed a nap. I felt old. After less than a week of being on the nutrition program, I have noticed an increase in my endurance and strength. No more naps. I don't feel tired. I am also sleeping better at night. I haven't taken a

stool softener either, no problem with hard stools. I am very pleased with these results, can't wait to see more."

Our final anecdote reveals how "AD" overcame both his insomnia and subsequent fatigue following his program designed using Nutrition Response Testing.

"My energy was low," explains "AD" (like many of my patients). *"I had a sluggish feeling. My sleep was often interrupted by general feelings of anxiety. My weight wasn't holding steady. My thinking wasn't very clear. I was on a mild antidepressant. Since being on the [Nutrition Response Testing] program, I have more energy. I have a generally lighter feeling. I've been off the antidepressants for about three months now. I am sleeping much better and my thinking is definitely clearer. My overall outlook is more accepting and positive."*

Don't let insomnia rule your life – or contribute to your fatigue. Seek help sooner rather than later. Experience the blissful feeling of whole-body wellness that becomes yours – forever – when you embark upon a personalized health improvement program based upon the safe, healthy and effective technology called Nutrition Response Testing.

Health Heist Handbook:

Few maladies are as frustrating as the battle between fatigue and insomnia.

Adrenal Exhaustion or Thyroid Fatigue
(A Case of Misdirection)

Some conditions extend beyond the scope of general feelings of fatigue, or even chronic fatigue and insomnia. "JB" was convinced that her previously diagnosed condition of adrenal exhaustion was the root of her illness. When I first saw her, she was confused, frustrated, in tears and at the end of her rope. Little did she know that her Nutrition Response Testing evaluation would soon provide the definitive path toward her experience of whole-body wellness:

"Before I began Paul Rosen's treatment plan [based on Nutrition Response Testing] two months ago, I was always exhausted, too thin, suffering from continual and seemingly random allergies to food and environmental substances. I felt like a limp rag after pushing my body to the edge of exhaustion with stressful work for many years.

"An ASI saliva test diagnosed me with Total Adrenal Failure Level 7, and a blood test showed a viral condition. My skin was thin, pale and slightly green. I was weak and unable to concentrate. I had to stop my exercise routine, and needed to rest in bed a great deal during daytime hours. I felt confused and desperate.

"My mealtimes were unpleasant, as my digestive organs contracted with pain frequently during and after mealtimes, as if they didn't want to accept what I was eating. My stomach remained full and bloated for three to six hours after mealtimes. I had eliminated many things from my diet, following an electronic allergy test. But my reactions did not agree with the allergy test, so I didn't

know what to eat and what not to eat. My bowels were irregular and too hard or too soft.

"For two months I have been following Paul Rosen's treatment plan and taking supplements with every meal. I have completely eliminated from my diet sugar, wheat, corn, soy and dairy. I added more protein to my diet, and eliminated most sweet fruits, as Paul Rosen suggested.

"Now after two months, I am not as tired and I can concentrate just fine. My food reactions are no longer random, they are extremely clear, and occur only if I eat any of the five things I am to eliminate from my diet. Mealtimes are pleasant and relaxing, as my digestive organs accept and digest what I eat. My digestion is still slow, but it is functioning. My digestion has stabilized. My bowels are regular once to twice per day, easy and clean.

"I have eliminated sugars from my diet, and I have no more sugar cravings. I have started to walk one mile three times a week. My circulation is improving and I have color in my skin. I feel physical stability in my life. I feel like I am in control of my health."

The reason what happened to "JB" is so important is because none of the standard saliva, blood and hair tests she took picked up the "missing piece" that would allow her body to begin the healing process. They failed her completely. In fact, these standard tests revealed a condition that wasn't even the real or root cause of her problem. Despite the assuredly caring efforts of many practitioners, both conventional and alternative, the diagnosis of "Total Adrenal Failure Level 7" given to her, while theoretically valid, failed to reveal that it was really her thyroid that needed attention.

With her body's stressors removed and proper diet and nutritional supplementation provided, "JB" fought her way back to health. Today she experiences the whole-body wellness that is part and parcel of balanced living. She found the "missing piece" – and so can you.

Stop living in isolation and fear. You are not necessarily the problem. It may well be that the diagnostic tests you and your practitioner assumed would reveal the answer fell short. And it only follows that the prescribed treatment program consequently fell short. In this way, even good treatments can fail. Some pieces of the puzzle are continually missed by the standard tests designed with a "one test fits all people" philosophy.

Does this sound far too familiar?

If you have even the slightest doubt as to whether or not you are experiencing whole-body wellness, I encourage you to get evaluated using Nutrition Response Testing. It's never too late to give alternative medicine a try. And why would you wait another minute to experience a better quality of life?

After all, in my humble opinion, it's not about how long we live. Rather, it's the quality of our experience with the time we're given on Planet Earth that truly matters. Ask those people who have witnessed their health deteriorate and then had it subsequently restored.

Health Heist Handbook:

"JB" was convinced that her previously diagnosed condition of adrenal exhaustion was the root of her illness. What she didn't know was that despite all the tests and clinical theory, her body could and would tell a different story.

Chapter 10

Painful Conditions

Few trials in this life are as disruptive as the appearance, and continuation, of pain. Be it frequent, severe, chronic or sudden, any type of pain immediately brings us to our own personal ground zero; it calls to mind our distant childhood, when life was lived in absolutes of black and white, happy or sad, joyful or fearful, painful or pain-free.

When pain appears in any body part, like the head, neck or back, or joints like shoulder, elbow, wrist or fingers, hips, knees, ankles or toes, whether or not these conditions are labeled as sciatica, arthritis, migraines or fibromyalgia, we become instant Neanderthals, forgetting our capacity for logic and reason, and act out of that most basic and primal humanoid reaction: relief.

In this state of "temporary insanity," we will grasp at *any* straw to relieve our pain. Liquid, powder, solid, capsule, whatever it takes: If the label gets our attention with snappy colors and the face of a smiling, pain-free person **and** promises us "speedy relief," we'll take it!

And, much like those early cavemen and cavewomen, we immediately start "hunting and gathering" the nearest pain remedies. Try watching less than an hour of television at any time of the day or night and count the contents of the few dozen commercials you see. No doubt a solid portion of those advertisements are for "fast," "quick" or even "instant" relief of a variety of pains.

The same can be said of our grocery, convenience, department and especially our drug stores. How many aisles – not shelves, but *aisles* – are reserved for "cures" for our pain? From aspirin to vapor rubs to portable heating pads to quick tabs to headache patches to oral toothache remedies to cushions to ease our foot pain, there truly is a "pill for every ill."

Naturally, your pain is "Big Business" to our friends in traditional medicine, in general, and to the pharmaceutical companies, in particular. According to the Joint Commission on Accreditation of Healthcare Organizations (JCAHO), "Overall, while the pharmaceutical market doubled to $145 billion between

1996 and 2000, the painkiller market tripled to $1.8 billion over the same period."

And according to the DEA, "… the increase in production of painkillers can be linked to the misuse or abuse factor. Although there is no precise statistic on how many persons misused or abused prescription painkillers, it is estimated that in 1999, four million Americans over the age of 12 used prescription pain relievers, stimulants or sedatives for 'non-medical' reasons."

As always, this chapter is in direct response to this distressing phenomenon. I want to show you **the alternative strategy for whatever kind of pain you're feeling**. Don't become a statistic and fall into the pain-medication trap. After all, there's a reason they're called "medications" and not "cures." (A more appropriate term might be "bandage" because all they really do is cover up the pain so that you can find some temporary relief.)

Nutrition Response Testing offers more than temporary relief. This exciting new technology actually (1) identifies the root cause of the problem and (2) provides a personal health improvement program that works. When you know better, you do better. Nutrition Response Testing helps you **know** better so that you can **do** better.

Health Heist Handbook:

We will grasp at any straw to relieve our pain. Liquid, powder, solid, capsule, whatever it takes: If the label gets our attention with snappy colors and the face of a smiling, pain-free person – and promises us speedy relief – we'll take it!

Headaches / Migraines

Anyone who has ever had a severe headache, let alone a migraine, knows that such pain can often be intense and, at times, even debilitating. The New York Times reported in an article dated August 8, 2006, that the World Health Organization (WHO) ranks migraines among the most disabling ills. Some 28 million Americans suffer with migraines while many millions more have them in milder forms. Employers lose the equivalent of $13 billion in lost productivity, with another $1 billion spent on medical care. All in all, statistics show that almost 18% of women and 6% of men experience migraines between puberty and 40 years of age.

Common triggers causing migraines are weather, missing a meal, stress, and alcohol and food reactions. A recent study shows that over half the sufferers consider crying to be a trigger. However, the bottom line is that, like most other symptoms, it is the autonomic nervous system reminding us that we are not heeding the warning signs.

Suppressive medication for migraines includes painkillers such as Imitrex, Zomig and Frova. These are triptans, and the use of these drugs requires active monitoring by a medical doctor because potential side effects, such as heart complications, can be severe.

Then there are the NSAIDS, or non-steroidal, anti-inflammatory drugs. An example of this group is Ibuprofen. Recent studies reveal serious side effects, including liver, kidney or stomach problems. In addition, they can cause rebound headaches. Soon, not only are you experiencing headaches from a source which is not clearly known, but you may also get additional headaches from the very drugs you take!

Some of you may have to resort to narcotics to ease your pain. The downside of these types of drugs is addiction. And last but not least are steroids. It is commonly known that the chronic use of steroids results in adrenal exhaustion, weight gain and chronic body pains – to name just a few. I once overheard a medical doctor say, "In these cases I have to decide whether to let my patient suffer with the disease he has or give him a different disease caused by the drug I prescribe."

Wouldn't it be amazing if all you had to do to ease your headache and migraine pain was identify and prioritize the five known stressors that can affect the healing process? (From Chapter 7: The 5 stressors are scars, food sensitivities, immune challenges, chemical challenges and metal challenges.) Relieve these stressors, provide whole-food nutrition and, voilà, migraines and headaches are a thing of the past.

This is what two people from our clinic had to say after starting their health improvement programs.

"HM" wrote of her success, *"I was getting four to six migraines per week; sometimes they came with really bad neck pain. After my first treatment, I noticed right away a decline in headaches. That first week after the treatment, I didn't have any headaches."*

Like so many of my patients, "HM" had been hesitant to give up or go without her over-the-counter pain relievers. But once she did, she realized the gift of true health had been waiting for her all along.

"I used to have a headache almost every day or every other day," wrote "RS" with relief. *"During the last five years or so I started experiencing migraines also. I had no idea what was causing them and was starting to get concerned that something serious might be wrong with me. I started on my program and within a week the headaches were gone."*

There are headaches that are severe and headaches that are chronic. Each has unique pain descriptors associated with it. "RH" suffered from both, but his chronic headaches became the reason for his first office visit.

"Before I came [to your clinic], I was in pain sometimes three weeks in a row with chronic headaches," he explained. *"Sometimes, I was even bedridden because of the pain. The only thing that would help would be to constantly take medications. After my appointments here, I instantly felt better. It has been a little more than three weeks and I haven't had a headache since. The program*

[identifying] the problem foods really helped and I can't think what it would be like without [that knowledge]."

"JH" had been a long-time sufferer of headaches, both severe and chronic, and was truly one of those patients who had his life given back to him by Nutrition Response Testing. Explains "JH" in his letter: *"I have had headaches since I was six years old. When I came here, I was taking six to eight Excedrin a day. There were many times that my pain would affect my entire lifestyle. My headaches now are almost gone. In the last two weeks, I have only taken six Excedrin. My energy level is much higher now and my attitude with my family is much better."*

"SH" had suffered pain ever since a traffic accident. *"I was rear-ended by a dumpster some 11 or 12 years ago. My neck is fused. Due to the pain and headaches, I have seen several doctors and specialists and have had a CAT scan and an MRI. Last fall I was going through several weeks of severe headaches and only three to four hours of sleep a night. After my third visit with Paul Rosen, the magic of healing without pills began. The treatments helped me beyond words. I am thankful to be able to be working again."*

Like so many of my patients, "RT" had gotten so used to having daily headaches that the pain was almost routine. *"I used to* have a headache at least once a day, usually upon arising in the morning," he explained in an email. "I would have almost instant diarrhea upon consumption of dairy products or leafy green vegetables. I have experienced radical improvement since starting the [Nutrition Response Testing] program. I haven't experienced a headache in three weeks now. I am now able to eat salads without deleterious effects. I have also lost 10 pounds in 90 days and have gone off Nexium and Allegra with no adverse effects."

Finally, "VP" wrote to tell me of her success with Nutrition Response Testing: "I was experiencing chronic pain between my shoulders and severe headaches (stress headaches) which were becoming increasingly frequent. My physician had prescribed Rizatriptan, which masked the pain but cured nothing. My massage therapist recommended I see an acupuncturist. My headaches are less severe and less frequent now. The pain between my shoulders is gone, and I've been able to do lots of yard work involving heavy lifting and pulling without re-injuring my shoulders."

If these stories sound too good to be true, ask yourself what's stopping you from seeking treatment like these patients. You don't have to suffer needlessly; relief is out there. I know trying something new can be daunting, but the point of these testimonials is to reach out a hand, to let you hear a familiar voice say that relief is available. You just have to find the "missing piece!"

Health Heist Handbook:

Anyone who has ever had a severe headache, let alone a migraine, knows that such pain can often be intense and, at times, even debilitating.

Arthritis

When it comes to both severe and chronic pain, arthritis is the rock star of my client's complaints. But they – and you – are not alone! Let's look at some statistics. According to the Centers for Disease Control and Prevention (CDC), arthritis is the leading cause of disability in the United States. The CDC has found that each year, arthritis impacts the United States with:

- 9,500 deaths
- 750,000 hospitalizations
- 8 million people with limitations
- 36 million ambulatory care visits
- 49 million people with self-reported, doctor-diagnosed arthritis
- $51 billion in medical costs and $86 billion in total costs

According to the National Institute of Arthritis and Musculoskeletal and Skin Diseases, more than 20 million people in the United States have the disease. By 2030, 20% of Americans – about 70 million people – will have passed their 65th birthday and will be at risk for osteoarthritis.

Younger people get osteoarthritis from joint injuries, but osteoarthritis is most often associated with older people. More than half of the population age 65 or older, both male and female, show x-ray evidence of osteoarthritis in at least one joint. Before age 45, more men than women have osteoarthritis, whereas after age 45, it is more common in women.

There is also rheumatoid arthritis, which is an autoimmune condition. The traditional theory for an autoimmune condition is that for some unknown reason the body is attacking healthy joints. However, I contend that the body is attacking itself for a **known** reason: because an irritant or stressor is affecting the joints and making them unhealthy. The immune system is simply trying to clear things up. And, to my thinking, this is why traditional testing methods often miss key information.

Conventional treatment for arthritis relies primarily on drugs. Surgery may be appropriate where a joint has degenerated to the point of no return. Such a joint (for example, a hip or knee) would be without articular cartilage or show severe degradation of bone. In these cases, replacement is clearly an option. However, the most important question to ask is whether such a condition is inevitable. I'm here to tell you that in most cases the answer is **NO!** Of course, where people have ignored the warning signs (like chronic joint pain), having a surgical option is a wonderful thing. But does that option work for every case? Obviously not.

Drugs are clearly so risky that it makes sense to look in other directions. It is now clear from recent recalls of drugs like Celebrex, Vioxx and many other painkillers that the dangers are too great. Even NSAIDS, those so-called "harmless" anti-inflammatory drugs you buy over the counter, can have life-threatening consequences such as kidney or liver failure. Before you automatically pursue a risky drug treatment, wouldn't it be worthwhile to first look at safe, natural and effective solutions?

Instead of seeking quick or "miracle" relief from expensive painkillers or serious surgery, find out the real cause and address it at the root in order to change the condition. Remember, with drugs, you are only suppressing the symptoms. You are only suppressing the pain. **YOU ARE NOT CHANGING THE DRIVING FORCE BEHIND THE CONDITION.**

Nutrition Response Testing is a technology that reveals the answers you seek. The sooner you act to discover the real cause, the less likely you will need radical intervention like surgery. What do you have to lose except some fundamental misunderstanding?

"HS" discovered Nutrition Response Testing as a last resort, and it was her best cure. *"I had experienced joint pain in most of my major joints for nine years,"* she wrote me not long ago. *"The location of the pain and degree fluctuated for no apparent reason. Traditional medicine had been unsuccessful in alleviating any of the pain and as a last resort I tried acupuncture. This worked better than traditional methods but was still not able to eliminate all of the pain.*

"Paul suggested a treatment of supplements using Nutrition Response Testing to determine the specific supplements needed. This, along with the acupuncture, has reduced my pain by about 80%. I am most pleased with the respect and concern shown during my treatments. When something did not seem to be working, I was considered the 'expert' and something new was tried. My experience with Western medicine was that if the treatment did not work, I was either blamed for not following instructions (not true) or my symptoms must be 'in my head.' This different approach was refreshing."

"SH" wrote to tell me, *"Thank you so much for your good work in helping me get well. After seeing you for acupuncture treatments, I am as good as new. No more hip or knee problems either. My husband Larry is doing well after his treatments, too! My daughter asked him, 'How did you get over your problem elbow?' Larry simply said, 'I had acupuncture.' He sounds like a true believer now. I really do appreciate your professionalism and your heart for helping others through healing techniques."*

Health Heist Handbook:

Nutrition Response Testing is a technology that reveals the answers you seek. The sooner you act to discover the real cause, the less likely you will need radical intervention like surgery.

Low Energy, Joint Pain and Digestive Discomfort

Low energy might not be considered "painful" to some, but ask long-time sufferers and they'll tell you that not having enough "get up and go" can be as deleterious as any of the painful discomfort we've discussed earlier, such as migraines and arthritis.

Take "EL" who, like many of us, wasn't a morning person. But his symptoms went much deeper. He explains, *"I had low energy. I was always tired in the morning. Now [after Nutrition Response Testing], I usually wake up refreshed. I feel good with less sleep. I have more energy also."*

Low energy can often be associated with digestive discomfort and when the two meet head-on, patients can be doubly uncomfortable. Such was the case with "LR," who complained, *"I had little energy and a lot of digestive discomfort. Herbs and acupuncture helped, but it constantly reoccurred. I also suffered with joint pain and backaches, along with neck pain. After beginning the [Nutrition Response Testing] program, I began to see major improvements. As long as I eat only the foods that I am allowed, I have little or no discomfort. I recently had a reoccurrence of symptoms and sought treatment. A laser light was used on both ear lobes and within two days – I felt great! I continue using herbs along with the occasional treatment in hopes that over time I will be able to adapt my life to constant healthy foods and little or no treatment."*

Like many patients, "DM" was experiencing low back pain as well as a variety of other maladies that all seemed related – and untreatable by traditional medicine. "DM" explains, *"I had little energy, felt run down, and had shoulder and back pain. My muscles and joints had aches and pains; getting out of the car was a chore. I was unable to run due to extreme lower back pain from the jarring. After just three days on the [Nutrition Response Testing] program, my shoulder pain was gone. Now, after two weeks on the program, my back pain has greatly decreased and I am able to run. I can get out of the car much faster and easier and don't feel like an old man when I do it. My muscles and joints feel much better. I have more energy. I am able to function at work at 6am, and the 10-hour days don't wear me out like they used to do."*

Some types of pain are more pronounced than others. Some come unannounced and unexplained. Such was the case with "CF" who found himself a pain-sufferer one morning. *"I woke up with severe rib pain on Tuesday, April 15th,"* he explains, recalling the very day his pain began. *"I couldn't sleep on my bed but had to sleep in my recliner. The pain kept me up during the night and was mild to intense during the day. [Acupuncture] treatments were given on April 21, 23, 25 and 28. On April 21, I was unable to take more than half a breath. After the initial treatment, breathing came back to about 80%. Subsequent treatment brought relief from pain. After April 28, I was once again able to sleep in bed. As of today (May 2, 2003), I am barely aware of any discomfort. I prayed that the Lord would heal me and I think he used Paul Rosen to accomplish this."*

"LS," like many patients, was more concerned for a family member than she was for herself. In this case, she brought her daughter in for treatment – and just in time!

"My daughter Sara, age 11, had stomach pain for over a year to the point of vomiting and uncontrollable shaking. The doctors diagnosed her with functional abdominal pain. After a year of sleepless nights and seeing my daughter in pain, we were not satisfied with this answer. A friend of ours mentioned her results from being on a [Nutrition Response Testing] program at Paul Rosen's office. It sounded a little 'out there,' but we were willing to try anything at this point...this program has been well worth it. After approximately one and a half months on the program, my daughter has had an incredible turnaround in her health, which is reflected in every part of her life. Her little vivacious attitude is back. She is able to sleep at night, no vomiting or shaking, and no pain in her

stomach. This happened gradually, but quicker than I had expected."

Sometimes pain leads to loss of sleep, which can, in turn, lead to low energy. Sometimes the reverse is true and lack of sleep and low energy lead to mysterious and painful symptoms. Such was the case of "LB," who wrote: *"I have chronic pain in my legs and hips, as well as extreme tightness in the muscles. After only one week on the [Nutrition Response Testing] program, I feel better. I am more energized when I wake up and the pain and soreness are not as intense as they used to be."*

Finally, an inspiring story from "BS," who wrote to express her relief after some digestive issues, which were affecting both her sleep and her job performance, improved. *"I used to take Ibuprofen and Aleve for pain and a prescription for digestive problems. I also took Lactaid to assist in digesting dairy products. I was only sleeping about three hours at a time because of the pain and digestive problems. Now [after Nutrition Response Testing], I take none of the above and sleep six hours at a time and sometimes nine. My stamina improves every day. I tutor at an elementary school, and am around lots of sniffles and sneezes, and haven't gotten a cold this spring. When my husband recently had the stomach flu for six days, I stayed healthy."*

I hope these successful client testimonials inspire you to find the "missing piece" to your own healing process and permanent relief from your painful condition. Whether it's chronic pain, isolated pain, post-surgical pain, pain from arthritis, digestive troubles or low energy, **any pain is too much pain**. We humans are designed to be pain-free. If you are experiencing more pain rather than less pain, you're simply not experiencing life fully.

Stop surviving – and start thriving. You can find the path to good health with Nutrition Response Testing. I firmly believe this, and I witness it every day in my clinic.

Health Heist Handbook:

Low energy might not be considered "painful" to some, but ask long-time sufferers and they'll tell you that not having enough "get up and go" can be as deleterious as any of the painful discomfort we've discussed earlier, such as migraines and arthritis.

Chapter 11

Digestive Conditions – With A Spotlight on Acid Reflux

Digestive conditions are now so common that they are experienced by millions of people each year. How many millions? Since there are so many digestive conditions (see the following list), it would give the author – and the reader – an "ulcer" (get it?) to track down the separate statistics on each and catalog them here.

Many digestive conditions are said to be inherited, or due to genetics. But when you look at genetics more closely, what health concern *isn't* related in some way to inherited genetic traits? The real question to ask is what triggers *your* genetic traits to manifest a health problem.

As it turns out, foods are one of those triggers. And, of course, most digestive upsets come from what we put in our mouths, whether it is liquid or solid. So, in a very real way, digestive conditions begin with poor eating decisions that rely on quick, convenient, fast, processed, zapped, fried or other "junk" food.

Environmental factors like chemicals, heavy metals and immune challenges (such as parasites) can play a role as well. And all digestive conditions are aggravated by stress and worry. Below are the most common digestive conditions I see – and successfully handle – in my practice:

- Acid reflux (so common that I've devoted a whole subsection to it)
- Bloating and discomfort after eating meals
- Digestive problems, muscle tightness, headaches and shaking
- Digestive problems with low energy
- Food allergies / diarrhea
- Anal itching
- Alternating constipation and diarrhea
- Stomach pain and canker sores
- Heartburn
- Excess gas and boating
- Water weight gain, skin breakouts and constipation
- Constipation
- Celiac sprue
- IBS

If you are suffering from digestive problems, I urge you to take them seriously because where there is smoke there is fire! "Little things" like indigestion or heartburn can denote "bigger things" like heart or thyroid complications. Warning signs like allergies, fatigue, bloating, diarrhea or constipation, when ignored or suppressed by drugs or herbs, can lead to or mask more serious diseases.

Pharmaceuticals and related suppressive therapies may provide temporary relief of symptoms, but the disease process proceeds unabated. Nutrition Response Testing is able to find the true root cause of these functional conditions and provide a health improvement program that enables the body's own innate healing power. In other words, put the most powerful healing tool on the planet– your body – to work by utilizing that amazing phenomenon I affectionately refer to as the "perpetual healing machine" and you *will* get well!

So many people suffer needlessly, like "T.I.", a former patient of mine. Her story is so similar to so many of my other patients' experiences that I wanted to relate it to you in full. Here it is:

"Before I came in to be evaluated, I spent the past six years trying to get healthy. My mom tells me that she can remember me having digestive problems even when I was two years old. I guess that means I've been suffering for a lot longer than six years. In fact, I don't really remember a time when I was actually· feeling good. I've tried going to numerous other doctors and have done years of research on my own, but I still continued to feel worse. I would always feel tired, bloated and had continuous diarrhea. I experienced excess sweating, which smelled awful. Not only that but I had allergies. Last year, whenever I cleaned my house, I would spend the entire day sneezing. My eyes would water and my nose would run the whole time.

"Most recently I worked with two naturopathic doctors. I spent six months with one and underwent allergy elimination therapy. The process even included some form of muscle testing. After [spending] a lot of money including [having to buy] multiple supplements, I saw very little improvement. I didn't know what to do or even where to go. Then one day I noticed that Mr. Rosen was to speak at a local health food store. I thought, 'What do I have to lose?'

"I went and was evaluated according to the Nutrition Response Testing protocol. After just one week on my program I saw positive results. Now, my diarrhea has pretty much gone. I'm beginning to feel energized after eating a meal instead of fatigue. At my evaluation my shoulder muscle was so weak I needed help to be tested. Now my muscle is strong. I just plain felt better. By the second week I could clean my entire house without a sneeze. No watery eyes or runny nose. I have not even had a hint of my seasonal allergies. In fact, I worked in my yard all day and had no allergy symptoms at all. I just couldn't believe how good I felt.

"One of the books Mr. Rosen provided explained the difference between synthetic vitamin supplements and whole-food products like Standard Process's. Now I understand why I wasn't improving. I would recommend that everyone read that book. In addition, I thought to myself, 'I wish someone had told me about this form of treatment long ago.' I would say, "Don't wait anymore. Get evaluated as soon as you can and get the improvement I got." I have so much more energy! I feel I can go to college, something I've always wanted to do but couldn't because I felt so sick all the time. Thank you Paul, Beth and Robin!"

Don't let digestive problems rule your life. Get to the bottom of them with Nutrition Response Testing. It doesn't matter if it's a big problem or a small one. Problems typically don't just go away. And, as we have seen, they can lead to bigger, more serious issues if left untreated.

Health Heist Handbook:

*Many digestive conditions are said to be inherited, or genetic. But when you look at genetics more closely, what health concern **isn't** related in some way to inherited genetic traits? The real question is what triggers your genetic traits to manifest a health problem. As it turns out, foods are one of those triggers.*

Acid Reflux

(Not Just Your Grandfather's Heartburn)

With so many digestive ailments presenting themselves to patients these days, I could write a book on digestive issues alone. However, one particular condition I do see more and more is acid reflux, and I want to address it specifically in a section of its own.

It is estimated that 5% to 7% of the global population, including infants and children, suffer from gastroesophageal reflux disease (GERD). Although common, GERD often goes undiagnosed because its symptoms are either downplayed or misunderstood. Left untreated, this condition can lead to serious complications, including scarring of the esophagus, and may increase the risk of esophageal cancer.

So how do you know if you have GERD and not something else? While you should be sure to check for a hiatal hernia first, persistent heartburn with acid reflux is the most frequent complication of GERD. Other symptoms include chest pain, hoarseness in the morning, or trouble swallowing. The backup of digestive fluids in the esophagus may also cause dry cough, bad breath and acid indigestion. However, it is possible to have this condition without experiencing *any* apparent symptoms.

Conventional Western medical treatment involves acid-suppressing drugs such as Prilosec, Nexium and Zantac. For advanced cases where there has been considerable damage to the body, surgery may be proposed. But in my experience: GERD began and continues to be a **functional disorder** – nothing more. And surprise, surprise! The overwhelming majority of my cases reveal the *real* cause of chronic heartburn to be too little digestive juices like pepsin (the protein-digesting enzyme) and hydrochloric acid. You heard me right! (We'll get back to this in a minute.)

Drug treatments, including the ever-popular over-the-counter antacids, are all about suppressing the warning sign – heartburn. Not only does this overlook the real cause of the disorder, but it is the basis for food allergies, bowel disorders and calcium-related problems including the compromise of our immune system. Some common conditions that may result include chronic fatigue (due to anemia), fibromyalgia, chronic sinus infections, IBS, celiac disease and osteoporosis.

For example, by shutting down hydrochloric acid production you shut down your body's ability to break down proteins and foods containing calcium. Incomplete breakdown of proteins can lead to larger than usual bits that, when absorbed in the gut, may be marked by your immune system as an "invader." Over a period of time, your body's defenders react to the slightest amount of these "bits," thereby creating food allergies. Food allergies are the basis of so many conditions like fatigue, chronic sinus infections and autoimmune disorders.

Calcium is important for, among other things, maintaining heart, muscle and bone health as well as for your immune system. Disrupt the body's proper calcium supply or calcium handling and trouble is around the corner. Shutting down the acid production of the stomach disrupts the proper breakdown of calcium-containing foods. For the body to be able to extract calcium, a highly acidic gut is crucial. Lack of bio-available calcium can lead to heart arrhythmias, muscle cramps, a weakened immune system and osteoporosis.

Okay, enough of the scare tactics. Like I said, acid reflux is a functional disorder. This means the autonomic nervous system is trying to tell you that an organ or a gland is not a happy camper. And over time nutritional deficiencies *will* compromise the proper function of the endocrine system.

Although we rarely think about them, the glands of the endocrine system and the hormones they release influence almost every cell, organ and function of our bodies. The endocrine system is instrumental in regulating mood, growth and development, tissue function and metabolism, as well as sexual function, reproductive processes and digestive functions. Yes, the endocrine system regulates stomach acid production.

Dr. Royal Lee observed that stomach acid regulation is related to the pituitary gland. Provide proper nutrition for the pituitary and magic happens. Of course, there may be other stressors involved, but a complete nutrition evaluation using Nutrition Response Testing will reveal the root cause of the problem. I have handled this functional condition successfully many times. Here is a story that is so inspiring I want to share it with you in its entirety.

"SR," a 51-year-old woman, came to my office complaining of a five-year history of acid reflux. She was a blonde woman, small and well-proportioned. She always appeared "just so" with make up and colorful clothes. She sat on the table and told a story that is a typical one in my clinic.

She began to experience indigestion, which gradually worsened. At first she tried to figure out which foods caused the problem. But even after discovering a few things, like tomatoes, she found no real pattern to her condition. The only thing she realized was that the condition was getting worse – and not better.

She began her medical intervention by visiting her doctor, who prescribed one drug after another, which either didn't work or worked to some degree but caused side effects she wasn't willing to live with. As each drug failed, she became more and more desperate. Feeling hope slip away, she had a conversation with her doctor's assistant, who told her about my clinic and Nutrition Response Testing.

As it turns out, "SR" put it off. (Sound familiar?) In fact, in her case she admitted that it was because she was "afraid to fail again." She felt that if Nutrition Response Testing failed she wouldn't know what to do next. It took over a year after first hearing of my work before she brushed aside her fears and finally got evaluated. Her result has been a blessing. Here is how she expressed herself:

"I used to go to bed with horrible heartburn. I would wake up with heartburn that would persist well into the day. I felt like I had swallowed acid. I would continually burp fire! Now, the heartburn is gone; even if I should eat before bed, I wake up without the upset stomach and raw esophagus.

"I suffered from acid reflux for at least five years. I went through all the medical tests and was given drugs. None of them worked very well. One that did caused horrible side effects. I didn't know what to do. My doctor's assistant told me about Paul Rosen but I waited over a year before seeing him. I was afraid that if what he did didn't work then what would I do? After being on my nutritional program for three months I rarely have any heartburn. The nice thing is that I now know what foods I am sensitive to so I have the power to avoid heartburn or reflux. I now have real hope that I won't have to live with this miserable condition."

Again, digestive conditions don't necessarily begin – or end – with acid reflux. Recall the veritable "laundry list" of concerns I listed at the beginning of this chapter, including bloating, food allergies and constipation among nearly a dozen others. Don't think that just because what you're feeling doesn't fall under this admittedly large umbrella Nutrition Response Testing won't work for you. It will.

All you have to do is get evaluated...

Health Heist Handbook:

Excess stomach acid is only a symptom identified with GERD. The underlying cause can be found in the recognition that GERD is a functional condition. It is your endocrine system crying for help. Let's check your pituitary gland for starters!

Chapter 12

Female-specific Conditions Featuring a New Look at Menopause (The Secret Revealed)

There's a great commercial on TV these days – and you know it must be good if I'm able to remember it – about one diet product or another. Now, I'm the farthest thing from an advocate for diet products, but it's the commercial that was potent enough to remember, not the remedy. At any rate, in the commercial a cartoon couple stands side-by-side; both the man and the woman are represented by drawings of two puffy, roundish-shaped people.

As the woman starts talking, she explains how her husband stopped drinking soda – and lost 12 pounds. Suddenly, the cartoon male shape in the commercial slims down! Then the wife explains how her husband stopped eating carbs, and lost 20 more pounds. Once again, the male shape slims down while the woman remains round and puffy. The punch line that always gets me is the woman saying, "And I haven't had a slice of bread in two years!"

I share this story to point out what I suppose the commercial was also trying to point out: Men and women are different: emotionally, physically, instinctively, biologically. Nowhere is this fact more evident than when it comes to various signs and symptoms that a woman may not be feeling as healthy as she should.

One way this difference is magnified is when talk turns to that of menopause, the big "M" word! How, exactly, does menopause affect women? According to the Mayo Clinic:

"Although your mother or grandmother may have used "the Change" to refer to menopause, it isn't a single event. Instead, it's a transition that can start in your 30s or 40s and last into your 50s or even 60s. You may begin to experience signs and symptoms of menopause well before your periods stop permanently. Once you haven't had a period for 12 consecutive months, you've reached menopause.

*"**Menopause is a natural biological process, not a medical illness**. Although it's associated with hormonal, physical and psychosocial changes in your life, menopause isn't the end of your*

youth or of your sexuality. Several generations ago, few women lived beyond menopause. Today, you may spend as much as half of your life after menopause..."

Symptoms and signs of menopause vary, but experts have come up with a quick list to portray the onset. According to the U.S. National Library of Medicine, "A woman has reached menopause when she has not had a period for one year. Changes and symptoms can start several years earlier." These include:

- A change in periods – shorter or longer, lighter or heavier, with more or less time inbetween
- Hot flashes and/or night sweats
- Trouble sleeping
- Vaginal dryness
- Mood swings
- Trouble focusing
- Less hair on head, more on face
- Yeast infections
- Chronic bladder problems

Let's be honest. Most women today fear menopause. They believe it will be the worst time of their lives, bringing unwanted symptoms like hot flashes, night sweats and sleepless nights, mood swings, panic attacks and osteoporosis. Who wouldn't be afraid? "Make it go away," women cry. And the wizards of Madison Avenue and the big pharmaceutical corporations – "Big Pharma" – hear you and promote it.

"Buy these drugs and it will be better," they say.

Is this scenario inevitable? Is menopause really a disease requiring drugs or surgery? What if the accepted explanation for a difficult transition through menopause is incorrect? What if the food we put in our mouths is the real culprit? Are there actually hidden health problems holding us back – and can they be successfully addressed using a holistic approach? What if a woman's mental and physical well being during menopause is really about attaining good overall health and not about treating symptoms?

In truth, menopause is (1) inevitable and (2) not a disease. I agree with the Mayo Clinic's viewpoint on this one. That said, menopause does not have to be a terrible experience. Once there were places on Planet Earth where the transition from childbearing years to menopause was seamless; no hot flashes, no night sweats, no heart disease and no osteoporosis.

These were places where women didn't eat processed sugar and foods containing preservatives, hormones, antibiotics, pesticides, herbicides and fungicides. They consumed whole, fresh foods and, interestingly, experienced little or no difficulty with menopause.

Women today hear from the medical establishment that menopausal symptoms are the result of too much or too little estrogen or progesterone. In addition, we're told that these two hormones play a major role in women's menses. Well, if this is true, it's important to note that synthetic chemicals (like the ones used to grow your food) are a major force creating significant imbalances in those two hormones – especially estrogen! For the whole sordid story, I suggest you read ***Our Stolen Future: Are We Threatening Our Fertility, Intelligence, and Survival? A Scientific Detective Story***, by Theo Colborn, Dianne Dumanoski and John Peterson Myers, with a Foreword by Al Gore.

It is no wonder women today may have hormone problems. Think back to your struggles with menstruation when you were young. What was your diet like? What chemicals were you exposed to? And what about now – years or even decades later? What exactly do you think is in those marvelous products you use on a daily basis for personal hygiene – perfumes, cosmetics, shampoos and conditioners, skincare products, body lotions, aerosol sprays, air fresheners, detergents and bathroom cleansers? You are being poisoned. And, like it or not – deny it or not, that old marketing adage "Better Living through Chemistry" is catching up with our generation and our children. Our health is at risk – and it won't go away unless we take action.

The number of women in this country undergoing hysterectomies rises every year. Following surgery, they are told they need "hormone replacement therapy" (HRT). This is medication containing one or more female hormones (usually estrogen and progesterone). But the truth is the ovaries are not the only source of estrogen production in the female body.

For all postmenopausal women, no matter how you got there, plenty of estrogen comes from adipose (fat tissue) and the adrenal glands. So, unless women have lost their fat tissue and adrenal glands, the persistence of symptoms is due to something besides hormone deficiencies. Fact!

Conventional medicine teaches that women struggle with menopause due to hormone deficiency. And over decades, medical doctors have been supplied with drugs provided by the pharmaceutical industries. These same drugs have finally been shown for what they are, hazardous to your health!

Then there are bio-identical hormones which, while possibly less risky, often miss the mark. Why? Because the overwhelming cause of hot flashes, night sweats, sleeplessness, anxiety, overactive bladder and so on is an **imbalanced endocrine system as a whole.** And this, too, is fact!

The endocrine system includes the ovaries as well as the pituitary, thyroid and adrenal glands. In my clinic, I successfully handle the most persistent menopausal cases by providing safe, natural and effective nutritional programs geared toward adrenal and kidney repair. **This is my secret revealed! FACT!**

Menopause is not a disease to be feared. It is a normal transition in the lives of mature women. If you struggle with symptoms, you need to know that hidden health problems are likely to be the cause of your distress and anxiety. Once you discover what they are, you can find relief *without* drugs and surgery. I know this and I am dedicated to making it known to others.

It's difficult to buck the "menopause fear" system. Especially since it was created by the conventional healthcare system you have been taught to rely on. However, if you are suffering symptoms *despite* doing everything your practitioner has recommended, you owe it to yourself to reexamine your assumptions.

I define insanity as doing the same thing while expecting to get a different result. It's just not possible. You have to make a change because any symptom, no matter how minor, should be heeded. The human body is not a "whiner;" it does not complain needlessly. When it's telling you something, it's best to listen. Find the "missing piece" in your personal health picture and enjoy a symptom-free transition through menopause.

Consider the story of "VP," who did experience hot flashes, found a food sensitivity using Nutrition Response Testing and well, let her tell you the rest:

"I had been feeling very well since beginning my [Nutrition Response Testing] program.... having eliminated back and shoulder pain, headaches, etc. But my hot flashes and night sweats were still a problem. One food that I really enjoyed and tended to eat too much of (snacking on them throughout the day) was cashews. After being

tested for and advised to stop eating them: Bingo! One day later my hot flashes had totally disappeared and have not returned."

Remember that this book is all about "stealing your health back." That includes not only paying attention to **your own body's signals,** but also to the results of your treatment. Question all the assumptions, including whether the hormone replacement theory is correct. If you're still experiencing any menopausal symptoms despite prior treatment, know there is a hidden health problem.

Another former patient of mine, "CJ," put it this way:

"I began to have severe menopausal symptoms starting about a year ago. The hot flashes during the day and the night sweats during sleep were terrible. I remembered how my mother suffered during her climacteric and how many years it took before she was over these problems. I asked my longtime acupuncturist, Paul Rosen, to help me lessen these menopausal symptoms. He started me on a [Nutrition Response Testing] program in which I use a special herbal treatment along with a diet plan. I began to feel much better within a week. The night sweats and hot flashes are pretty much gone and I sleep comfortably every night..."

Keep in mind, however, that while I've shared with you two very common testimonials about menopause and related symptoms, they are *not* the only female-specific condition that can be remedied with Nutrition Response Testing. The following list represents just some of the more common female conditions I handle successfully in my clinic on a daily basis:

- Infertility
- Yeast infections
- Weight control
- Skin conditions
- Menstrual irregularities
- PMS
- Menopausal symptoms
- Chronic bladder problems

My point in writing this chapter is to make you aware that a dominant viewpoint is not necessarily the best or even correct one. There are safe, natural and effective alternatives. But to get different results you require a different viewpoint. If you're still experiencing any symptoms despite prior treatment, know there is a hidden health problem and find it with Nutrition Response Testing. You, too, can become an advocate for health improvement in this country, starting with your own.

Health Heist Handbook:

*Remember that this book is all about "taking your health back." That includes not only paying attention to **your own body's signals** but also to the results of your treatment. Question all the assumptions, including whether the hormone replacement theory is correct. If you're still experiencing any menopausal symptoms despite prior treatment, know there is a hidden health problem and find it!*

Chapter 13

Respiratory Conditions

Among the many causes that result in the umbrella event known as "respiratory conditions," allergies are usually the ones you hear the most about. "Allergy" is a term that refers to many conditions such as drugs, "bugs" and foods. The category I'm most interested in here is seasonal allergies rooted in food sensitivities.

True food allergies, where an individual consumes a peanut, for example, which results in a life-threatening condition called anaphylactic shock, affects a very small group of people. It is estimated that 1% to 2% of adults are affected by *true* food allergies. However, a much larger group of people, both adults and children, suffer from the more common "food sensitivities."

Reactions include sleepiness after eating, irritability, stuffy nose, runny eyes, acid indigestion, bloating, pain and swelling of the joints as well as weight gain, to name just a few. Over time these can lead to seasonal allergies, asthma, IBD, chronic fatigue and a variety of immune disorders.

Discovering whether or not you have food sensitivities can provide not only dramatic relief from unwanted symptoms but may very well prevent serious disease. **Nutrition Response Testing is a technology for discovering if food sensitivities are the underlying factor hindering your body's health improvement.** Here is what others have said about their allergies, both before and after experiencing a Nutrition Response Testing program:

- *"I used to have bad seasonal allergies. I would be on antihistamines for a majority of the spring and summer. This year is my third spring without a single antihistamine. I'm able to enjoy being outside and active without being dragged down by antihistamines."*

- *"I had been experiencing GI irritation and significant anal itching. I tried to do various dietary things to alleviate the irritation from this embarrassing symptom. I tried reducing grains and flours and this worked randomly. Paul [Rosen] applied Oriental medicine and Nutrition Response Testing and came up with allergies to egg whites, soy and oats. I had been consuming a lot of these foods on a daily basis to increase my protein. After a week of eliminating egg whites, soy and oats, that embarrassing symptom was gone. If I have something with oats, the symptoms come back that same day. I have experienced marked improvement for well over three months now."*

• *"Before Nutrition Response Testing, my health was what I would have called good. I just accepted my problems because I'd lived with them my whole life and assumed everyone else was the same. I had a lot of digestive problems, low energy levels, and an immune system that didn't seem to work very well because I often caught cold and flu viruses. However, now I am highly aware of what I put into my body and how it affects it. I can tell almost immediately when I've eaten something I shouldn't have. I have more energy than I had before. My digestive problems have gone away for the most part, and when I start to get sick I know what to take to get rid of the virus before it takes hold. I feel like I'm on the road to healing."*

Of course, just as menopause isn't the only female-specific condition we talk about in Chapter 12, please don't think seasonal allergies are the only respiratory condition addressed by Nutrition Response Testing. In my experience, all of the following are handled routinely in my clinic:

- Acute/chronic colds and flu
- Sinus problems

- Chronic cough
- Runny nose
- Watery eyes

It's common to hear mainstream physicians say that there is nothing people can do to treat colds and flu. Yet I see clients all the time who learn to handle both colds *and* flu by following their personalized health improvement programs. This is what Bethany had to say:

"I used to get sick a lot. I always seemed to feel like I had a cold or flu. I just seemed to feel sick all the time. This sick feeling seemed worse whenever I ate. When I got my personalized health improvement program I began to see quite a bit of improvement.

"However, at some point my improvement stopped. I felt better than worse. When Paul pointed out that I might have a [personal] relationship impacting my health, I knew immediately who it might be. I began to address the problem. Once a plan was in place, the next time I saw Paul I reported that my health took a huge leap forward. I began to make additional progress. I feel better physically and emotionally. Food tastes so much better and there is no sick feeling. I have more energy than ever before."

You have to keep in mind when reading about or listening to health issues in the media (or anywhere for that matter) who is doing the studies. Where does the money come from for these studies and what are the motives behind the scenes? The FDA, the AMA, and the pharmaceutical companies are so closely tied that it can be difficult to know where one begins and the other ends. Keep a healthy skepticism and, as they say: Just follow the money!

My clinical experience (like that of hundreds of other alternative practitioners who utilize Nutrition Response Testing technology) shows that people like you and me can either avoid the flu completely or recover from it quickly using alternative strategies. Say what you will, when a healthcare strategy utilizing good solid nutrition works over and over, turning away from it is like turning your back on yourself. It's a crying shame, and I'm quite serious.

I have treated many people with conditions similar to Bethany's and have witnessed the same excellent results. I am not being self-serving when I urge you to find yourself a practitioner who knows Nutrition Response Testing. My mission is to do all I can to give people the tools they need to regain a healthy body. I searched long and hard to find the "missing piece" to my own health dilemma and those of several of my family members. We have benefited enormously from our experience and wish the same for you.

Health Heist Handbook:

Discovering whether or not you have food sensitivities is the first step to discovering the root cause of seasonal allergies. Once accomplished, you will find all the hold-ups preventing you from experiencing high-quality respiratory health.

Chapter 14

Emotional Conditions

Have you ever heard the expression "a dog's life"? People use it in an envious fashion, perhaps today more than ever, to point out how easy dogs have it. Run, fetch, sleep, dream, eat, run and fetch some more. And don't forget sleep!

As humans, we don't quite have this luxury. While our thoughts, inspirations, hopes and emotions separate us from animals – dogs, cats and everything in between – they can make life endlessly complicated if left to their own devices.

Our emotions and thoughts can be powerful and uplifting, inspiring us to reach new heights and accomplish goals no mere animal could ever hope to achieve. They provide us with literature, song, romance, love, laughter and passion. Too often, however, our emotions get the best of us, resulting in prolonged states of anxiety, insomnia and even depression.

But do we have any control over our emotions? If so, what can we do to gain or regain control when we're overwhelmed? It is true that our attitude has an effect on our health. But it is also true that our endocrine system has a lot to do with emotion generation and harmony.

Ladies and gentlemen, it's all about the hormones.

If your endocrine glands are struggling and poor nutrition predisposes them to malfunction, then you may very well find yourself overcome with emotions. For example, fear and anxiety are connected with the health of our adrenal glands. Irritability and anger are related to the thyroid gland. Organ health plays a role, too.

Joy and despair are associated with the heart, guilt and sadness reflect the lung and worry and obsession mirror the digestive organs. These are functional relationships observed for thousands of years and reflected in Oriental medicine. There is a balance to be had, which rests to a great degree upon what we put in our mouths and what we are exposed to in our environment. These are the hidden health problems.

Like so many of our emotions, anxiety is both a blessing and a curse. According to the National Institute of Mental Health (NIMH), "Fear and anxiety are part of life. You may feel anxious before you take a test or walk down a dark street. This kind of anxiety is useful – it can make you more alert or careful. It usually ends soon after you are out of the situation that caused it."

What if it doesn't go away? What happens when anxiety becomes less useful – and more all-consuming? "For millions of people in the United States," concludes the NIMH, "the anxiety does not go away, and gets worse over time. They may have chest pains or nightmares. They may even be afraid to leave home."

The line between a healthy level of anxiety and an unhealthy one is thin, and personal. Only you can know what feels "comfortable" for you, but I caution you to pay careful attention to this "thin anxiety line." Remember, the body is not a whiner and your high anxiety is most likely the reflection of a hidden health problem.

"KE" is a patient who found increased levels of anxiety to be a major concern. Like so many sufferers of deep and persistent anxiety, he suffered from multiple conditions. In his case, these conditions included chronic pain, sinus infections and digestive disturbances. These concerns, combined with the already persistent state of anxiety he'd been living under, had a ripple effect that had him seeking professional help. I'll let him explain:

"When I came to see Paul I was having a lot of anxiety and heartburn plus muscle pain, joint pain and sinus infections. I was taking Intermax minerals and Airborne and there were no changes.

Since I have been coming to AcuNatural Family Healthcare I have no more anxiety, heartburn, sinus infections or muscle pain and surprisingly, the liver spots on my skin are gone too. There is a 95% improvement in my joint pain. AND as an added bonus I have lost 35 pounds. Now, when I have a hard day at work it takes about a half of a day to recover when it used to take a couple of days."

Like so many other patients suffering with emotional conditions, "KE" blamed his condition on stress. But life *is* stressful, right? His daily stress did not change a bit and yet, with the proper health improvement program, his debilitating conditions melted away. So don't be misled. Stress is not the sole enemy. By getting the tools you need to gain control of your emotions, you will find your world changing dramatically.

Much like anxiety, stress can be both positive and negative. According to the NIMH: "We all have stress sometimes. For some people, it happens before having to speak in public. For other people, it might be before a first date. What causes stress for you may not be stressful for someone else. Sometimes stress is helpful – it can encourage you to meet a deadline or get things done. But long-term stress can increase the risk of diseases like depression, heart disease and a variety of other problems."

Pay attention! If you feel yourself breaking down under the stress, look around and make changes if you can. Delegate or drop a few activities. Take time for yourself, and include physical exercise and some form of contemplation. But be aware that poor nutrition is by far the most important factor you must face. **Fact!** Beneath it all, poor nutrition is the "2,000-pound rhino" in the room, and you have to do something about it. You owe it to yourself and to your family.

How much stress is too much? The answer is quite personal, but I think sharing this story from a female patient named "CB" might help:

"I am 34 years old and was battling a deep depression. I had broken down and after seven years decided that I would get drugs to treat my illness. My medical doctor instantly prescribed an antidepressant after seeing my Beck Inventory score of 39, the

highest score he had seen in five years. I took my first pill and upon arising the next morning could not function. I was extremely faint, dizzy and super nauseous. My head hurt and I was crying. I am thankful for this experience because I knew I didn't want to live with negative side effects my whole life. The next day I came to see Paul [Rosen]. I knew I had to try acupuncture again, as it was what saved me three years earlier from depression. After my acupuncture treatment, Paul told me about [Nutrition Response Testing].

*"I started the program after being tested sensitive to soy, wheat, sugar and dairy. Two days later, I left on my prescheduled vacation at the beach for four days. I was very diligent at taking my supplements and stayed away from all the foods that were found to be bad for me. By the time I returned on Saturday evening, I felt 95% better! Even after returning to normal life, getting up at 6am to fix my husband's lunch and getting my 11-year-old and 7-year-old off to school at 8am and starting my day with my 4-year-old and 1 ½-year-old, I still felt 80 – 85% better than I had just one week earlier. While on vacation, I had the book Paul had given me, **Going Back to the Basics of Human Health**.*

"That book helped solidify that sugar is not in my future and that gave me extra strength to 'Just say no to sugar!' I went back to my medical doctor three weeks to the day after he prescribed drugs. He could not believe how great I looked and felt. He asked how I liked the other drug he gave me samples of and I told him I never tried it. I told him about NRT and acupuncture and he was glad to see me so much better. He had me take the Beck Inventory test again and I scored "0"!!! Don't let another day go by before having a [Nutrition Response Testing evaluation]. The #1 thing I have noticed is that my hundreds of negative feelings and thoughts are GONE!! Thank you, Paul, and thank you, God!"

The thing I love about this story is how much it says about "CB" as a person. I am grateful to her for acknowledging me as part of her recovery, but the truth of the matter is her success was dependent upon her willingness (1) to be open to something new and (2) to follow through with the recommendations. Without these two things, neither "CB" nor anyone else would benefit from what was clearly the blueprint for her success.

Remember, **you can't get healthy – or stay healthy – if you are not involved**. I am not here to knock your medical doctor or traditional medicine. I am here to offer a point-counterpoint evaluation of the various disorders and ailments discussed in Part 2 of this book so that you know there is a choice – **and the choice is up to you**.

Health Heist Handbook:

Like so many other patients suffering with emotional conditions, "AD" blamed his condition on stress. But life is stressful, right? His daily stress did not change a bit and yet, with the proper health improvement program, his debilitating conditions melted away. So don't be misled – stress is not the sole enemy. Get the tools to gain control and your world will change dramatically.

Chapter 15

Cardiovascular Conditions

If any area of health exemplifies intentional confusion, it's the complicated – and confusing – subject of heart health. The study that set the basis for the lipid hypothesis of heart disease was done in the 1950s. The doctor who performed these studies in Russia was David Kritchevsky. As a reminder, the lipid hypothesis claimed that heart disease resulted from eating saturated fats and the cholesterol found therein. It stated that foods like meat, dairy and eggs were harmful and should be avoided. It likewise stated that margarine and vegetable oils, which contain poly-unsaturated fats, were preferable.

Now, I'd like to take this hypothesis to task. First of all, note that the Kritchevsky studies were done on rabbits, which are herbivores not carnivores. Yet the rabbits were fed animal products. If that isn't enough to call into question whatever the good doctor's results would show, then subsequent studies have seriously questioned the hypothesis itself.

For an unbiased look at the history of this issue, I invite you to read **Diet & Heart Disease**: *It's Not What You Think* by Stephen Byrnes, Ph.D., RNCP. Another great source of unbiased information is "The Oiling of America" by Sally Fallon and Mary Enig, published in Australia's *Nexus Magazine* (Dec/Jan 1998, Feb/March 1999). And when I say unbiased, I mean sources with no connection to the government, pharmaceutical, medical or food industries.

In the second place, the human body requires saturated fats in order to properly utilize essential fatty acids. In his book, Stephen Byrnes writes: "Saturated fats lower the blood levels of the artery-damaging lipoprotein (a), elevate HDL levels, are needed for proper calcium utilization in the bones, and provide a good energy source for vital organs. They stimulate the immune system, protect the liver, do not initiate free radical formation and are non-irritating to the arterial walls. Omitting them from one's diet, then, is poor advice." (Page 50)

Thirdly, Byrnes goes on to say: "Cholesterol is needed by the body to manufacture an array of hormones, as well as contribute to the structural integrity of the cell wall. Cholesterol is also needed for the proper function of serotonin receptors in the brain. Serotonin is what makes us 'feel' good; this is why low cholesterol levels are associated with higher rates of depression, suicide and aggressive behavior. Dietary cholesterol plays an important role in maintaining the health of the intestinal wall...Cholesterol is also needed for the proper development of the brain and nervous system...Despite this and the fact that low fat diets cause learning disabilities, stunted growth and failure to thrive, major public organizations recommend low fat/cholesterol diets for children!" (Pages 50-51) And the health risks for adults are documented as well.

The Framingham Heart Study, touted for its support of the lipid hypothesis, has been characterized by several experts in this way:

"In Framingham, Massachusetts, the more saturated fat one ate, the more cholesterol one ate, the more calories one ate, the lower people's serum cholesterol...we found that the people who ate the most cholesterol, ate the most saturated fat, ate the most calories weighed the least and were the most physically active." (William Castelli, M.D., Director, The Framingham Study – see The Weston A. Price Foundation for source).

"The diet-heart hypothesis has been repeatedly shown to be wrong, and yet, for complicated reasons of pride, profit and prejudice, the hypothesis continues to be exploited by scientists,

fund-raising enterprises, food companies and even governmental agencies. The public is being deceived by the greatest health scam of the century." (George Mann, SsD, M.D., former Co-Director, The Framingham Study – see Weston A. Price Foundation for source).

"An analysis of cholesterol values…in 1,700 patients with atherosclerotic disease revealed no definite correlation between serum cholesterol levels and the nature and extent of atherosclerotic disease." (Michael DeBakey, M.D., pioneer of heart transplant surgery – see The Weston A. Price Foundation for source).

Finally, *"The relevant literature [on coronary heart disease (CHD)] is permeated with fraudulent material that is designed to convert negative evidence into positive evidence with respect to the lipid hypothesis. That fraud is relatively easy to detect."* (Russell L. Smith, Ph.D., author of an authoritative study on CHD – see The Weston A. Price Foundation for source).

When I initially started reading information like this contradicting the established "facts" we'd been taught, my world was turned upside down – and I'm sure, reading this, yours is, too. But the bottom line, and I tell you from my own experience, is this: **Avoid polyunsaturated fatty acids (PUFAs), the kind found in vegetable oils like canola and corn. Instead eat plenty of pure**

butter and cold-pressed oils like olive, coconut and sesame. With the addition of grass-fed meats, including beef, pork and lamb as well as poultry and fish, eggs and raw dairy products, you have the diet your healthy ancestors ate not that long ago!

Nutrition Response Testing will reveal the nutritional basis for handling many conditions associated with heart health. These include:

- High blood pressure
- Fatigue
- Irregular heartbeat
- High cholesterol
- Arthritis
- Shortness of breath
- Leg cramping during sleep
- Restless legs

One of the biggest concerns I see in my clinic, and the one I'll spend the most time detailing in this chapter, is high blood pressure. High blood pressure is as common as indigestion these days. It is a condition worthy of the pharmaceutical industry's lust. Granted, there are certain situations that are referred to as "primary hypertension." But this is a rare disorder of the arterial system of the lung. Only 500-1,000 cases per year are diagnosed. The condition appears mostly in women ages 20-40, but anyone from children to adults can be affected.

Secondary hypertension affects a smaller group of people, approximately 5% of those with high blood pressure. These conditions are also related to another organ or gland, like a kidney or thyroid, which is malfunctioning.

The majority of high blood pressure cases are those of unknown origin, which seem to relate to lifestyle conditions such as obesity and diet among others. Regardless, since nutrition and dietary factors are primary to overall health, Nutrition Response Testing has proven to be effective in handling secondary hypertension and the majority of cases whose origin is unknown.

Dorothy, age 59, was placed by her medical doctor on medications for high blood pressure. She was overweight but not obese. She then experienced the drugs' side effects, including fatigue, numbness in her feet, dry eyes and flaking skin. Her concern was to not have to live with long-term medications.

Because of her willingness to make the minor lifestyle changes necessary to avoid the side effects of her blood pressure medication, she went to her medical doctor regarding the drugs. We then put her on a personalized health improvement program using the Nutrition Response Testing technology. This is what she said soon thereafter:

"I had high blood pressure, recorded at 186/96 and climbing. I had low energy and was tired all the time. After one week of starting the program, my blood pressure was recorded at 137/82. My energy improved. I'm not so tired even though I was getting less sleep due to working the night shift. Now I mentally want to get up and get going and exercise!"

And Dorothy reported an additional benefit: weight loss or, in her words, "three belt notches."

Please understand that high blood pressure, along with many of the body's symptoms we might experience, is one of the "check engine" lights of the autonomic nervous system. The implication is that "the marshal" controlling your bodily functions is not very happy. Medications only suppress these "check engine" lights, they do not address the underlying cause.

Suppression in these cases is similar to glancing down at the dashboard of your car only to find a "check engine" light gleaming in the dark. You decide to pull off the road and reach underneath to pull the wire to that light. With the "check engine" light ignored, you drive off down the road only to experience an inevitable breakdown. Of course, you would never do such a thing, right? But it's like this: When you address the root of the problem, not only does your blood pressure begin to find its balance, but many other conditions resolve themselves as well.

Robbie had this to say after starting her Nutrition Response Testing program:

"Due to circumstances in my life over which I have no control, my life is more stressful than I can ever remember. Because I am following Paul Rosen's directions, in spite of the stress, I have felt better, slept better, my mind works better and is clearer. I have lost 10 pounds and have started a walking exercise program again. I have heart problems, and my heartbeat has been more regular and my blood pressure checks out normal."

Even when we are under emotional stress, if we feed our bodies the proper whole food nutrition we will be able to handle that stress – period.

Health Heist Handbook:

You must understand that high blood pressure, along with many of the body's other symptoms, is one of the "check engine" lights of the autonomic nervous system. The implication is that "the marshal" controlling your bodily functions is not very happy. Medications only suppress these "check engine" lights, without addressing the underlying cause.

Chapter 16

Skin, Hair and Nail Conditions

Are you satisfied with the quality of your skin, hair and nails? Are you proud to walk out of the house, feeling radiant and looking great? Do you have a regular routine and a healthy system in place to make sure that your skin, nails and hair look, feel and actually are their best?

Or are your skin, nail and hair concerns so deep and profound that they have become a serious issue for you? Are they affecting your social life – or how often you leave the house? Or even how comfortable you feel about your appearance and health when you *do* leave the house?

If you are one of the many modern Americans who fall into that second group, you might be suffering from one or more of the following skin, nail and hair conditions I treat daily:

- Dry spots on face and arms
- Acne
- Psoriasis

- Eczema
- Dry skin
- Itchy scalp

- Brittle nails
- Dry/thinning hair

Unfortunately, people have a tendency to write off concerns like those I've listed as simply cosmetic or "surface" issues. In point of fact, nothing could be further from the truth. Remember those "check engine" lights I mentioned in the last chapter? You know, the ones that, if ignored, could spell doom and gloom along your journey down Life's physical highway?

Well, blood pressure and heart problems aren't your body's only "check engine" lights. Often enough, troubles on your body's surface like dry skin, itchy scalp or brittle nails are pointing to something deeper and more serious.

"HH" was suffering with a severe acne problem when he came to see me recently. Here is how he described his resulting recovery from a condition he once feared might be life-long:

"I had severe acne problems with my facial skin. I have never had such bad acne in my life, not even as a teenager. I recently met

with my dermatologist. He prescribed doxycyclene, an antibiotic, which basically makes the skin "appear clear," as he put it. I took the horse pills for at least four months (three refills). My skin cleared up a little, but not enough for all the medication I was consuming. My dermatologist told me if I wanted clear skin I just needed to keep taking this prescribed medicine. I decided I did not want to live on drugs for semi-clear skin and stopped visiting my dermatologist. My mother recommended I see Paul Rosen. Now [after Nutrition Response Testing] 80 % of my acne is gone without taking doxycyclene. I have also noticed an increase in my energy level. Since starting with [Nutrition Response Testing], I have improved greatly in less than a month."

"NG" feared his problems with itchy scalp might dog him for the rest of his life, too. That is, until he tried Nutrition Response Testing:

"From November to March for three years, I was having diarrhea after I ate. At first it was only in the morning. I had a very itchy scalp unless I took fish oil capsules everyday. For the past six

years my fingernails were cracking, splitting, and getting worse. Taking calcium with magnesium, a multi-vitamin plus eight other herbs didn't help. I would also awaken each morning after only four to five hours of sleep, and then would have trouble falling back to sleep again. My energy level was very low after 5pm. My doctor or a naturopath could not seem to help. Now after five weeks of avoiding wheat, sugar, corn and dairy, I am doing much better. The diarrhea stopped immediately. My scalp stopped itching, and the ridges on my nails are less pronounced. I sometimes can sleep longer than five hours. My energy is good now until 8pm. Here are the other benefits I am getting without looking for them: no more sinus trouble in the winter, no more itchy skin, less anxious, and a growth in the corner of my eye fell off after I happened to rub my eye."

"CE" had raging psoriasis for 18 years. His body was 85% covered with bleeding sores that itched mercilessly. Over the years, he used topical ointments, UV treatments and drugs, including Methotrexate and Amevive. While he did get significant symptomatic relief, the side effects and costs were overwhelming. Amevive alone cost over $14,000 per year!

So, at the urging of his wife who had experienced success with her own personalized health improvement program, "CE" came for an evaluation. He said:

"After beginning my program, I saw dramatic relief in three weeks. The psoriasis had all but disappeared. I was still doing the UV treatments but decided to stop them. In the past, stopping my UV treatments would result in reemergence of my symptoms, but not this time. I was ecstatic!"

As a postscript, "CE" related that during a visit to his dermatologist, when he flashed his new skin, the attending nurse said to him, "We've never lost a patient because they got better!" Need I say more?

Like "HH," "NG," and "CE," you too may be feeling insecure or worried about your skin, nail and hair problems. Don't be! The beauty, fashion and cosmetics industries have been doing a number on us for years. We've become so insecure about our appearance that we use their hyped lotions, creams, soaps, shampoos and so on, all expensive and loaded with chemicals, while few of them actually produce noticeable results.

That is because true beauty starts within, and I'm not being touchy-feely here. I'm talking about real, true, natural and physical beauty starting from what you eat, and how you live your life. These are qualities you gain by learning to listen to and understand your body, and trusting Nutrition Response Testing.

Health Heist Handbook:

They say beauty is only skin deep. Maybe, maybe not. But one thing is for certain: If you are suffering with skin, hair and nail problems, there is a deeper health concern. Find it, treat it with proper nutrition and you will look and feel better and Better and BETTER!

Chapter 17

Eye, Ear, Nose and Throat Conditions

Nutrition Response Testing holds out hope for a variety of conditions. Which of those conditions are the most important? The answer, like so much of Nutrition Response Testing's best results, rests squarely with you. For instance, if brittle nails are your biggest problem, than that is the most important symptom I can help you with. If it's high blood pressure, than that's the most important condition – to you.

So it goes with the eye, ear, nose and throat conditions I see quite often, two of the most popular being runny nose and watery eyes. In fact, "SL" is a typical patient in this regard, as you'll soon see.

" For 30 years I have dealt with allergy symptoms including runny nose, watery eyes and headaches. To make matters worse, I also experienced TMJ, upper back pain, stiffness and tiredness.

In the past, I have spent tens of thousands of dollars going to every type of doctor and alternative healthcare professional imaginable. Although some of the conditions improved, as I aged, they were still bothering me. There has been a notable improvement now that Paul has helped me isolate the "stressors" on my system and really pinpoint my chronic hyperthyroid condition as the culprit behind most of my physical complaints. My health is improving weekly and I have made a major life-style change which I know will benefit me and give me the quality of life I have been searching for."

We have a tendency to discount so-called "lesser symptoms" such as runny nose and watery eyes. But if you've ever dealt with them on a persistent or even casual basis, you'll know firsthand that they're anything but. Take your nagging cough, for instance. Not long ago, a patient we'll call "TS" presented us with this very symptom, which at first started as a nuisance but might have been a sign of something more serious if she had waited much longer to schedule an appointment:

PAUL J. ROSEN, J.D., L.AC.

"I was coughing and blowing my nose so many times a day I thought I should invest in the Kleenex Company. I was driving my husband and co-workers crazy! I went to work tired everyday. I wanted to go right to bed as soon as I came home from work. I could sleep Saturday and Sunday until noon or 2pm. Now [after Nutrition Response Testing] I can breathe and not cough! I don't have post-nasal drip! I get up feeling refreshed and I have energy all day. This has changed my life in just seven days. I have also lost two pounds!"

Please heed the message that **no** symptom is more important than any other. In "TS's" case, a nagging cough was just that, a nag that was easily remedied. But in other cases I've seen patients complain, almost apologetically, of similar symptoms that turned out to be much more serious than at first indicated.

The best part about Nutrition Response Testing is that it's more than just a method for evaluation; it provides you with a lifestyle fit for you. I don't just have patients. I have relationships. Why do you think I'm able to include so many personal testimonials on these pages? My patients become passionate about living a new lifestyle, one that is personal and created specifically for them. This is not "medicine by numbers." It is a custom-designed treatment program for individuals who need it – and it changes their lives drastically for the better.

Health Heist Handbook:

We have a tendency to discount so-called "lesser symptoms" such as runny nose and watery eyes. But if you've ever dealt with them on a persistent – or even casual – basis, you'll know firsthand that they're anything but.

Chapter 18
Male-specific Conditions

In our chapter on female-specific conditions, I focused mainly on menopause (the "M word"). In my chapter on male-specific conditions, I'm going to dwell on the prostate (the "P word"). But what exactly **is** the prostate?

According to www.prostate.com, "The prostate is a gland of the male reproductive system that produces fluid for semen, which helps to transport sperm during the male orgasm. The prostate is made up of about 30% muscular tissue; the rest is glandular tissue. Normally, the prostate is small—about the same size and shape as a walnut. It is located in front of the rectum and just below the bladder. The prostate wraps around the urethra, which is the tube that carries urine out from the bladder through the tip of the penis."

Problems with the prostate run the gamut from enlarged prostate to erectile dysfunctions, all of which are potentially serious.

According to the National Kidney and Urologic Diseases Information Clearinghouse (NKUDIC), "6.5 million of the 27 million Caucasian men 50 to 79 years of age in the United States were expected to meet the criteria for discussing treatment options for BPH (benign prostatic hyperplasia, or enlarged prostate)."

Pretty much every older male knows that the most common prostate-related symptom is a restricted urine stream. But (and here is the point of this chapter) there is a symptom that is a most commonly *unknown* prostate-related problem and that is chronic low back pain. This chronic low back pain is often experienced in combination with neck, upper back and shoulder pain, too. You heard me correctly, and it's so important that it bears repeating: **If you are a male suffering with chronic low back pain, check the prostate.**

My patient "DM" was quite surprised that his evaluation at my clinic revealed nutritional deficiencies with his prostate reflex. He was kind enough to recount the following:

"I had little energy, felt run down, and had shoulder and back pain. My muscles and joints had aches and pains; getting out of the car was a chore. I was unable to run due to extreme lower back pain from the jarring. After just three days on the [Nutrition Response Testing] program, my shoulder pain was gone. Now, after two weeks on the program, my back pain is greatly decreased and I am able to run. I can get out of the car much faster and easier and don't feel like an old man when I do it. My muscles and joints feel much better. I have more energy. I am able to function at work at 6am and the 10-hour days don't wear me out like they used to do."

Prostate problems can become quite serious if left untreated. And while the traditional medical establishment says that 50 is the standard age recommended for men to start getting checked for prostate problems, many of my patients can recall experiencing low back pain as early as their teens.

I am here to tell you that if you give your body the right nutrition, things will turn around. The prostate is like every other organ and gland in our bodies: they all require the right nutrition to correct any deficiencies. I guarantee that if you are suffering discomfort in your body, there is a deficiency somewhere. Nutrition Response Testing listens to the body and translates its needs to us. That's the simple part. The hard part is for a person to finally decide to listen to their body's needs and to take action.

Health Heist Handbook:

The most commonly known prostate-related symptom is a restricted urine stream. But did you know that chronic low back pain is equally common? This low back pain is often experienced in combination with neck, upper back and shoulder pain, too.

Chapter 19

Neurological Conditions

Neurological conditions are so common and so profligate that I could write a book on them alone. How common? According to the National Institute of Neurological Disorders and Stroke (NINDS), "More than 600 disorders afflict the nervous system. Common disorders such as stroke, epilepsy, multiple sclerosis, Parkinson's disease and autism are well known. Many other neurological disorders are rare, known only to the patients and families affected, their doctors, and scientists who look to rare disorders for clues to a general understanding of the brain as well as for treatments for specific diseases. Neurological disorders strike an estimated 50 million Americans each year, exacting an incalculable personal toll and an annual economic cost of hundreds of billions of dollars in medical expenses and lost productivity."

Such a huge quantity of disorders, many of them severe, makes a catchall chapter (like this last one in my book) quite a challenge. But, as with all things emotional or physical, it boils down to the "patient of one" **You**. What is *your* disorder? What are *your* symptoms? How do they affect *your* health, *your* hope, *your* present and *your* future?

A kind woman, PR, wrote me to explain how Nutrition Response Testing helped her overcome her diabetic neuropathy and subsequent loss of balance:

"When I started with Mr. Rosen, I was taking three medications twice a day for diabetes, one for high blood pressure and one for thyroid. My blood pressure was always something over 90 or above, and my blood sugar levels were always high in the morning, sometimes normal [but] mostly elevated during the day. I have had pain in my feet for years and spider veins around my ankles and have been overweight most of my life.

"One of the things that I noticed was that when I closed my eyes and was standing up, I would loose my balance. [Since being on my nutrition program] the biggest change in this short period of time is the change in my medications. I now only take one diabetes pill a day instead of two. I have stopped taking blood pressure medication altogether. My blood pressure readings are between 123-140 over 79-85. This is much better than it was when I was taking the medication. I have not been falling over lately because my balance is better. I find I have more energy. The purple veins on my ankles are now going away and I have more feeling in my feet."

It might surprise you that Nutrition Response Testing can affect something as serious sounding and imposing as a neurological condition. However, after all, **the body is the perpetual healing machine!** In other words, the body knows only two states: balance or imbalance. Other conditions that my colleagues and I successfully handle:

- Tremors

- Multiple sclerosis

- Carpal tunnel

If you read back over the previous chapters in Part 2 of this book, you will see that a lack of balance is at the heart of our bodies' malfunctioning. In PR's case, her lack of physical balance reflected a disruption in the body's homeostasis. But in every case noted in this book, a "lack of nutritional balance" is at the root of the problem. This is true whether it is a woman's body or a man's, whether it is a young body or old, whether the symptoms are brittle nails or an enlarged prostate.

When the body is out of whack, it lets us know. That is why we must be in tune with our own body's "check engine" lights such as muscle weakness, numbness, twitching or shaking, high blood pressure, frequent urination, heightened anxiety or hot flashes.

We do our bodies a great disservice when we give too much importance to certain symptoms, like the brain or the heart, and not enough to others, like the skin and hair or the ears, nose and throat. To me, all symptoms are serious. That's because with Nutrition Response Testing we evaluate the body as a whole and not just the "biggest," "best" or "most important" parts.

The sooner you stop thinking of your body as Kentucky Fried Chicken (that is, a pile of pieces and parts, some more important than others), the faster your hidden health problems will be discovered using Nutrition Response Testing – and the sooner you will feel better.

Health Heist Handbook:

*If you read back over all of the chapters in Part 2 of this book, you will find **a lack of nutritional balance** at the root of the various conditions introduced; whether for women or men, young or old, symptoms of brittle nails or prostate-driven low back pain.*

Epilogue

Hope for the Future; Help for the Now

So here we are, at the end of our journey together – but also at the beginning of another journey. By this I mean your personal journey toward a safe, natural and effective restoration of your health through Nutrition Response Testing.

Now, in the final analysis, I sincerely hope that this book has inspired you. **Hope**, after all, was the reason for its inception; results were reasons for its completion. It's easy to get caught up in all the medical jargon and legal mumbo-jumbo out there. But when pain is present, we tend to grasp at straws. When we are suffering, we're willing to gamble and spend any amount of money on a whim, a hot tip or a rumor. As they say, "A pill for every ill."

But with just the little bit of knowledge we've shared together, hopefully now you can see there is a better way. There is a safe, natural and effective way to recapture your health from those who stole it from you. Don't be misled: "Big Pharma", the processed food industry and the unwitting medical establishment are ready, willing and able to steal it back again if you fail to take control.

The simple and wonderful truth is that the human body is a miraculous system designed for self-help, self-control and self-regeneration. It is a remarkable perpetual healing machine, willing to respond if and when we're willing to listen.

It's time to reexamine the way we examine health, our own and that of society at large. By adding Nutrition Response Testing to your methods of evaluating your health concerns, you've added the technology of the future, and you've done it today. When you receive a personalized health improvement program from someone trained in Nutrition Response Testing, get ready to be amazed. You will be in awe of "the skin you're in" and what it can tell you when you know how to communicate with it.

So much of our pain is self-inflicted. I know it's not nice to hear, but how do you think your body feels about it?!? The way we eat, the pace we maintain, the stress we put ourselves under, the junk we feed ourselves, the poor decisions we make – especially regarding what we put into our mouths, all of these things serve to throw our bodies out of whack. We are, in every sense of the word, our own worst enemy. Think about it.

But now that you know better, you can do better. This book that I call *The Great Health Heist* is less about *who* stole your health (the "heist" part) and more about what *you* can do to get it back (the "great health" part).

So often in life we play the blame game to the point of injuring ourselves in the process. What can we do about big corporations, really? How can we stop the glut of pharmaceutical products that come down the pike annually? What can we personally do about the rows and rows and aisles and aisles of "a pill for your ill" products that crop up each year?

"Nothing," you say. Try again. There *is* something you can do, and it starts with *you*. Stop buying into the hype and **start questioning your assumptions**. "What assumptions?" you ask. I'm talking about assumptions like these: (1) that if the drugs you take mask your symptoms, then your health must be good; (2) that it's okay to treat health concerns with toxic drugs rather than by nourishing your body with the right whole foods and whole food supplements; (3) accepting the established protocol that blood, bowel, saliva, hair and skin tests reveal all there is to know when evaluating a health concern (just remember how often such tests find nothing wrong); (4) that consuming just a little bit of sugar and processed foods is harmless; and finally (5) accepting that you have no control over your own health.

The first word in self-help is "self" because *you* have to be the one to *help* yourself. This book reveals a simple and effective option, and that's what so many of my patients say as their health improves and they get off drugs. "I wish someone had told me about Nutrition Response Testing years ago" is the common refrain.

The only thing that sends a message to doctors, advertisers, and the chemical, food and pharmaceutical industry is money; when they start losing your money, they *will* change. So get started now!

If it still sounds too daunting, don't think of it in medical terms – think of it in movie terms. That's right. We all complain about the lack of quality in today's movie theaters: the violence, drugs, sex, inanity, lack of plot, loud explosions – the list goes on and on. But why does Hollywood keep making the same movies over and over again? There's one reason – they continue to make money. Our complaints go unheeded because they know we find it easier to just sit through another bad movie on date night rather than actually spend quality time with our date! So until we actually do the one and only thing Hollywood fears – and that is stop buying tickets to their cruddy movies, they will continue to make cruddy movies.

You don't need an MBA to figure that one out. And you don't need a medical degree to realize that traditional medicine and the big pharmaceutical companies will stop ripping you off once you put your foot down and stop buying their products.

Still skeptical? When I came across Nutrition Response Testing, I was very skeptical, too. That surprised Dr. Freddie Ulan, considering I'm an acupuncturist, where placing needles in people is supposed to relieve pain. But look how it has changed my life, look how it has changed the dozens of patients' lives who have graciously shared their testimonials in this book. I'm passionate about this subject because I know it can change your life, too!

You're scared? It's okay to be scared. We've relied on our aspirin, our sleep aids, our antacids, our uppers, our downers, our caffeine, our alcohol, our pills and tubes and creams and lotions and potions for so long, we wouldn't begin to know what to do without them. But I know – you'll finally start to live again!

Just make one change and, I promise you, the other changes will get easier and easier. It's your body – for life. You don't get another one and there are no trade-ins. If you know something's wrong with you and it seems just a little too easy that a single blue or pink or green or purple pill will "make it all go away," then guess what. You're right! If you play the game of drugs, you lose!

But you have the power. You don't have to contribute to *The Great Health Heist* any longer. You don't have to buy into the lies, the deceit, the myths and the fables – and you certainly don't have to buy any more products that won't work, can't work and are destined to leave you worse off than you were before.

All you have to do is try something new. That's really it. Just try.

Aren't you worth that much?

I know you are and your body knows you are. Now you have to believe that you are, too. I think you're ready. Know why? You're still with me! How many pages have you stuck with this? How many testimonials do you need before you write one for yourself? How many statistics, anecdotes, stories or quotes do you need before the message hits home? Hope is out there.

And the best part is, it's available *now*. It exists. You don't have to wait for government approval or the price to go down or the supply to increase or the methods to perfect themselves. The results are in: Nutrition Response Testing works.

But only if you give it a try…

Health Heist Handbook:

The Great Health Heist *is less about who stole your health (the "heist" part) and more about what you can do to get it back (the "great health" part). Now you have an option.*
Get evaluated today!

SOURCES

BOOKS

- Dr's Joseph Mercola and Kendra Degen Pearsall, *Sweet Deception: Why Splenda, NutraSweet, and the FDA May be Hazardous to Your Health,* (Nashville, TN: Thomas Nelson, Inc., 2006)

- Ray D. Strand, M.D., *Death By Prescription: The Shocking Truth Behind An Overmedicated Nation,* (Nashville, TN: Thomas Nelson, Inc., 2003)

- Thomas L. Friedman, *The World Is Flat: A Brief History of The Twenty-First Century,* (New York: Farrar, Straus and Giroux, 2005)

- Sally Fallon w/ Mary G. Enig, Ph.D., *Nourishing Traditions: The Cookbook That Challenges Politically Correct Nutrition and the Diet Dictocrats,* (Washington D.C.: NewTrends Publishing, 1999, 2001 2nd Revised Edition)

- Stephen Byrnes, Ph.D., RNCP, *Diet & Heart Disease: It's NOT What You Think...,* (Warsaw, IN: Whitman Publications, 2001)

- Henry G. Bieler, M.D., *Food Is Your Best Medicine,* (New York, N.Y., Ballantine Books by Random House, 1966)

- Dr. Bernard Jensen & Mark Anderson, *Empty Harvest: Understanding the Link Between Our Food, Our Immunity And Our Planet,* (New York: Avery [Penguin, Putnam, Inc.] 1990)

- Dr. Edward Howell, *Enzyme Nutrition: The Food Enzyme Concept,* (New York: Avery [Penguin, Putnam, Inc.] 1985)

- Joel Salatin, *Holy Cows & Hog Heaven: The Food Buyer's Guide To Farm Friendly Food,* (Swoope, VA: Polyface Inc. 2004, 1st Edition)

- Weston A. Price, D.D.S., *Nutrition and Physical Degeneration,* (Weston A. Price, 1939, 1945 then La Mesa, CA: The Price Pottenger Nutrition Foundation, Inc., 1970-2004, 6th Edition)

- Nancy Appleton, *Lick The Sugar Habit,* (Garden City Park: Avery Publishing Group, 1996)

- Mary Frost, M.A., *Going Back To The Basics Of Human Health: Avoiding the Fads, the Trends and the Bold-Faced Lies,* (San Diego, CA: Dist. By International Foundation For Nutrition And Health, 1997-2004, 3rd Edition, 2004)

- Harvey W. Wiley, M.D., *The History of a Crime Against The Food Law,* (Milwaukee, WI: Lee Foundation For Nutritional Research, 1955, original publication by Harvey Wiley, Washington D.C., 1929)

- Marcia Angell, M.D., *The Truth About the Drug Companies: How They Deceive Us and What To Do About It*, (New York: Random House, 2004,2005)

- Doris J. Rapp, M.D., *Our Toxic World: A Wake Up Call* (Buffalo, NY: Environmental Medical Research Foundation, 2003, 2005)

ARTICLES/LECTURES

- Dr. Royal Lee, *Vitamin News, 1933-1956,* (Fort Collins, CO, Selene River Press)

- Dr. Royal Lee, *The Triad: Dr. Royal Lee and the Immune System, presented by Mark R. Anderson,* (Fort Collins, CO, Selene River Press, 2004)

- David Morris, DO, *Royal Lee, DDS: Father of Natural Vitamins,* (article www.westonaprice.org/nutritiongreats/lee.htm)

- Dr. Royal Lee, *Lectures of Dr. Royal Lee Volume I (1940-1963),* (Compiled by Mark R. Anderson, Fort Collins, CO, Selene River Press, 1998, 2000)

- Dr. Royal Lee, *Lectures of Dr. Royal Lee Volume II,* (Compiled by Mark R. Anderson and Stephanie Selene Andersen, Fort Collins, CO, Selene River Press)

- Dr. Royal Lee, *An Introduction To Protomorphology,* (International Foundation for Nutrition and Health)

- Dr. Royal Lee and John Courtney, *Conversations in Nutrition,* (International Foundation for Nutrition and Health, 2001)

- NY Times, Science Times, pub. 4/3/07, *Drugs are in the Water: Does it Matter?*

- "The Oiling of America" by Sally Fallon and Mary Enig, published in Australia's *Nexus Magazine* (Dec/Jan 1998, Feb/March 1999)

WEBSITES

- *www.TheGreatHealthHeist.com (Where to order this book)*
- *www.acunatural.com (Paul's home website)*
- *www.mercola.com*
- *www.wikipedia.com*
- *www.westonaprice.org*
- *www.realmilk.com*
- *www.price-pottenger.org*
- *www.ifnh.org*
- *www.diabetes.org*
- *www.drugs.com*
- *www.nytimes.com*
- *www.cdc.gov/nccdphp/aag/aag_arthritis.htm*
- *www.standardprocess.com*
- *www.prostate.com (click on 'about the prostate')*
- *www.unsinc.info*

About the Author

Paul J. Rosen, J.D., L.Ac.

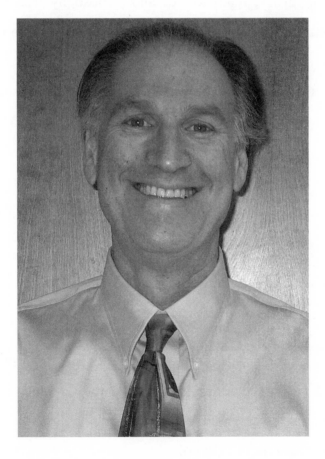

Paul J. Rosen, JD, LAc, is a licensed acupuncturist in Portland, Oregon, and Vancouver, Washington, where he is clinic director of AcuNatural Family Healthcare. A Detroit native, he graduated from Western Michigan University with a bachelor's degree in chemistry, mathematics and philosophy. He holds a law degree from Indiana University School of Law-Bloomington and was a trial attorney in Boston for seven years before deciding to pursue his interest in alternative healing methods. He subsequently attended Emperor's College of Traditional Oriental Medicine in Santa Monica, California, graduating with distinction and a master's degree. Traditional Oriental medicine includes the disciplines of acupuncture, herbal medicine, tui na (massage), and dietary and nutritional therapies among others.

Following postgraduate work in Shanghai, China, where he earned a certificate of achievement, he underwent specialized acupuncture training in Stans, Switzerland. He then studied with Dr. Richard Tan, a master and founder of the "Balance Method" of acupuncture, and presented papers at Dr. Tan's 2002, 2003 and 2004 conferences in San Diego.

212

Mr. Rosen's most recent achievement is in the field of nutrition where he is a certified advanced clinician of Nutrition Response Testing. In his clinic, established 14 years ago, he is dedicated to health improvement program design as opposed to the conventional "symptom management" model followed by Western medical practitioners. His studies with Freddie Ulan, DC, CNT, and Lester Bryman, DC, CDN, founders of Nutrition Response Testing, have enabled that goal, and Drs. Ulan and Bryman call on him to train other doctors and healthcare practitioners around the country.

His popular call-in radio show called "Health Matters with Paul Rosen" airs regularly in the region. He has appeared on Portland/Vancouver network and community television (KATU-ABC, FVTV) and been interviewed on several radio stations. As an advocate for organic foods and local farmers and farmers' markets, Paul frequently gives public talks at Wild Oats and Whole Foods Markets in Portland and Vancouver. In addition, he holds free workshops regularly at his clinic and makes himself available as a speaker to interested groups.

Paul Rosen's AcuNatural Family Healthcare clinic is located at 306 East 37th Street in Vancouver, Washington, just across the mighty Columbia River from Portland, Oregon. His mission and that of his enthusiastic clinic team is to provide clients with a true and proven alternative to drugs and surgery. For information on his clinic and practice and current and upcoming events, visit his website: www.AcuNatural.com or call (360) 750-7375. For information about his book and where to purchase it, go to www.TheGreatHealthHeist.com.

How To Get Evaluated

The Great Health Heist is less about who stole your health (the "heist" part) and more about what **you** can do to get it back (the "great health" part). Now you have an option. Get evaluated today.

So go to www.TheGreatHealthHeist.com to find a link to a list of qualified health care practitioners. Pick one in your area who will identify the "missing piece" to your health puzzle putting you on the path to restoring the quality of your life. Don't wait; take back your health today!

Be sure to share what you've learned in this book with someone you care about.

To order a copy go to www.TheGreatHealthHeist.com.

6-20-23